Dear Reader,

Unnoticed and unsung, healthy hands perform countless small tasks, from pouring your morning coffee to brushing your teeth at night. But aching hands transform even a simple task into a painful ordeal. Beneath the skin, your hands are an intricate architecture of tendons, joints, ligaments, nerves, and bones. Each of these structures is vulnerable to damage from illness or injury. Arthritis can make it difficult to carry a shopping bag. Carpal tunnel syndrome can interfere with your work and hobbies. Hand or finger deformities can complicate basic daily routines such as getting dressed.

Hands are also a tool of communication, expression, and emotion. Because a person's hands are nearly always visible, people tend to be very conscious about the appearance of their hands, and hand pain or deformity can cause embarrassment and inhibition, triggering feelings of poor self-esteem.

In this report, you'll learn about the major problems that afflict hands. Your hands may hurt for a variety of reasons, from the mechanical to the neurological. Persistent joint problems such as arthritis—which affects one in five American adults—are by far the most common cause of hand pain and disability. This report describes the many different forms of arthritis and ways to relieve arthritis-related hand pain, from use of assistive devices (tools and other gadgets that take strain off your hands) to medications and surgery. And although the prevalence of these disabling conditions is on the rise as the population ages, advances in artificial joint replacement hold promise for easing the pain and loss of function for people with severe forms of these diseases. A Special Section addresses joint reconstruction for arthritic hands.

Injuries to nerves and tendons also cause problems. Carpal tunnel syndrome affects an estimated 2% to 3% of Americans. Contrary to conventional wisdom, this nerve disorder rarely results from repetitive work-related tasks. Regardless of the cause, there is help in the form of medication, splints, hand therapy, and surgery. Other highlights of this report include the latest treatments for common tendon injuries and an evolving nonsurgical treatment to ease a disabling hand problem known as Dupuytren's contracture.

Finally, you'll learn how to avoid the most common hand injuries, including sprains, fractures, and amputations—and you'll learn how to keep your hands healthy and strong so you can enjoy the pleasures of work, play, communication, and expression for years to come.

Sincerely,

Barry P. Simmons, M.D.
Medical Editor

Joanne P. Bosch, M.S.P.T., C.H.T.
Medical Editor

The healthy hand

It's hard to imagine getting through a day without using your hands. Beyond their countless practical functions, like opening doors, eating, and driving, we use these complex structures in many other ways, to both convey and perceive information.

People who can't speak or hear use their hands to converse through sign language. But even hearing people often use their hands to communicate—by throwing them in the air in frustration, by applauding, or by touching someone's shoulder. You may clench your hands in anger or clasp them together in prayer. Your hands can even offer clues to your personality (consider the impact of a warm, firm handshake).

People who can't see use their hands to read, thanks to the exquisite sensitivity of the fingertips. Although your sense of touch spreads all over your body, your hands are the main organ you use to gather tactile information about your environment.

Hand structure and physiology

Because the hands perform many functions, it's no wonder they have a complicated design (see Figure 1, page 3). Sadly, complexity can also lead to trouble.

Bones. Each of your hands has 27 bones. Together, the 54 bones in your two hands make up a quarter of the total bones in your body. However, their number and proximity means that if one thing goes wrong, it can also affect nearby parts of the hand and wrist.

Muscles, tendons, and ligaments. To control movement, each hand has 34 muscles, which are found in the palm and forearm. About a quarter of the brain's motor cortex (the part that controls all movement in the body) is devoted to the muscles of the hands. But surprisingly, there are no muscles in the fingers—only ligaments and tendons.

Tendons in the hand connect muscles in the forearm to bones of the fingers and thumb. When a muscle contracts, it pulls on the tendon, which then pulls on the bone and moves it. Flexor tendons, on the palm side of the hand, help you bend or flex your fingers, while extensor tendons, on the back of the hand, help you straighten them. An entire chapter of this report is devoted to tendon troubles.

The remarkable human thumb

You may have heard that an opposable thumb is one key anatomical difference that distinguishes humans from animals. Actually, many animals—including chimpanzees, koalas, and even opossums—have opposable thumbs, which means they can oppose, or touch, the thumb to the index finger. But humans have a unique ability to also oppose other fingers to the thumb, thanks to flexible joints in those digits. It's this ability that allows you to strongly grip and grasp objects. About 40% of the hand's function is attributed to the thumb.

Opposable thumbs that can touch all the other fingers give human beings great dexterity.

Other thumb facts

- The word thumb comes from the Latin tumere, meaning "to swell"—a nod to its short, thick form.
- Because of the shape of its joint, the thumb can move in a larger circular pattern than the other fingers.
- The slight hollow on the dorsal (top) side of the wrist at the base of the thumb is known as the anatomical snuff box, so named because snuff (powdered tobacco) could be put there and inhaled.
- Also referred to as the first finger or pollix, the thumb has three bones (two in the thumb itself and one that connects it to the wrist). That's one fewer than the other fingers.
- People who are born without a complete thumb or who lose one in an accident can undergo pollicization—the surgical creation of a thumb from a finger, usually the index finger. Another option for replacing a lost thumb is a toe-to-thumb transfer.

While tendons attach muscle to bone, ligaments bind bone to bone, holding the bones together and keeping them in proper alignment. The ligaments on either side of your finger joints prevent excessive side-to-side deviation, while the ligaments that stretch across your palm keep your fingers from bending too far back. The job of stabilizing the joints goes to both ligaments and tendons.

Both tendons and ligaments consist of tough connective tissue fibers made of collagen, the protein that gives them the strength and flexibility to perform their distinct functions. Because these fibrous tissues have little blood supply, however, tendon and ligament injuries heal slowly.

Tendons in the hand are largely covered by protective sheaths that resemble deflated balloons. The inner lining, or synovium, produces a clear, slippery fluid resembling egg white, called synovial fluid. (In fact, the word synovium comes from the Latin term for "with egg.") The joints, too, are lined with synovium

Figure 1: Inside the hand

Under the skin, the hand's 27 bones and 34 muscles work in synchrony to perform a range of movements, from a powerful hammer blow to a gentle caress.

Bones

Muscles and nerves

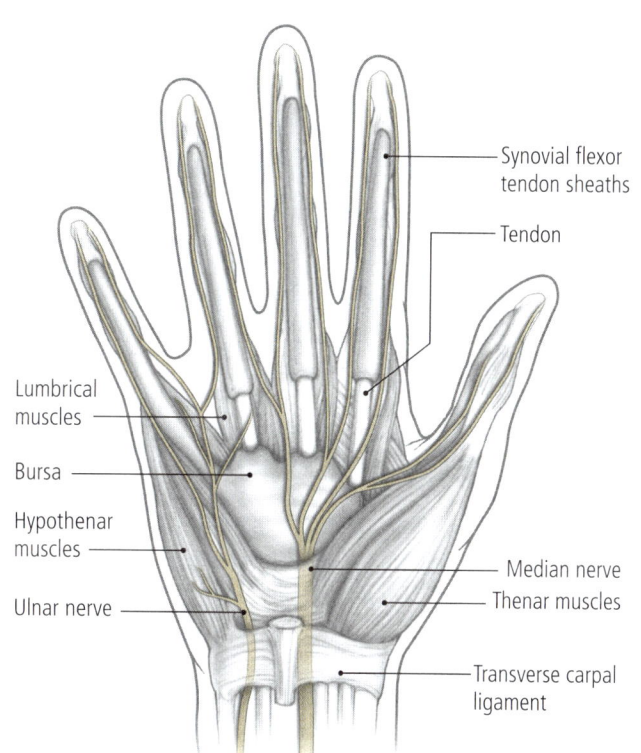

The main bones of the hand are the metacarpals, which connect to the finger bones, or phalanges. The knuckle joints that connect these bones are the metacarpophalangeal (MCP) joints. Each finger has three phalanges and the thumb has two. The middle joint of the finger is the proximal interphalangeal (PIP) joint. The joint near the end of the finger is the distal interphalangeal (DIP) joint. Instead of DIP and PIP joints, the thumb has one interphalangeal (IP) joint. The major bones of the wrist are the carpals, which connect to the ends of the larger forearm bones, the ulna and radius. The carpals connect to the metacarpals at the carpometacarpal (CMC) joints.

The small but powerful muscles of the hand are located entirely in the palm and forearm. The fingers have no muscles. Fingers are controlled by tendons attached to the muscles of the hand that help to flex and extend them. Two major nerves are the median nerve (leading to the thumb, index, and middle fingers and the inner half of the ring finger) and the ulnar nerve (leading to the small finger and the outer half of the ring finger). The bursa helps cushion the hand.

and filled with synovial fluid. This vital substance lubricates tendons and joints, providing frictionless movement of the fingers. It also supplies nutrients to nearby bones and cartilage.

Cartilage. This tough and somewhat elastic tissue cushions joints and provides a smooth, slick surface for movement. When it degrades, this leads to osteoarthritis, one of the leading problems in the hand.

Nerves. Three major nerves (the radial, median, and ulnar) serve the hand. The median nerve, which passes through the wrist, is noteworthy because pressure on this nerve causes carpal tunnel syndrome.

The nerves in your hands also gather crucial information about the world around you and enable you to react swiftly. For example, why can most people instantly withdraw their hand when their fingers touch a hot object? The credit goes to a complex sensory system, including closely packed nerve endings in the skin, connective tissue, and joints of the hands that detect pressure, light touch, vibration, joint position, heat, and pain. These receptors relay information through the peripheral nerves and spine to the somatosensory cortex of the brain, where the input is processed and messages sent to the motor cortex for response. If nerves are cut or compressed, the system is disrupted, diminishing the ability to distinguish between touch, pain, and changes in pressure and temperature and to tell where the sensations are coming from.

The nerves are also essential for things like gripping and pinching, which depend on hand and wrist position, forearm and hand muscles, and the positioning of fingers. Grips are divided into several types, depending on the position of your thumb and fingers: power grip (with fingers flexed toward your palm, as when grasping a suitcase handle); cylindrical grip (wrapping thumb and fingers around an object but not touching each other, as when holding a drinking glass); and fist grip (wrapping thumb and fingers around an object, as when holding a hammer or squash racket). Pinches are divided into two major types: three-point pinch

---

How a certified hand therapist can help

A certified hand therapist is either an occupational therapist or a physical therapist who has specialized education and training in rehabilitation of the hand. This specialist evaluates your hand's range of motion and strength, as well as any pain, swelling, or physical limitations caused by your condition. He or she then applies a wide range of therapies to help you regain normal use of your hand. Common conditions that may warrant seeing a hand therapist include arthritis, tendinitis, carpal tunnel syndrome, or trigger finger.

A hand therapist may give you exercises to increase your strength and range of motion.

A hand therapist's toolkit includes such varied treatments as massage, heat or ice applications, ultrasound to warm and increase blood flow to muscles and joints, and iontophoresis—a technique in which an anti-inflammatory medication is driven into the skin using a low-dose electrical current. Another treatment, called fluidotherapy, uses a machine filled with tiny particles of cellulose, which are suspended in a heated stream of air, creating a whirlpool effect. Gently exercising your hands within the warm chamber has a soothing effect. The therapist can also help relieve pain and stiffness by dipping your hands in warm paraffin wax melted in an electric appliance that maintains a safe temperature. After the wax hardens, the therapist wraps the treated area in a plastic sheet and blanket to retain the heat.

Do not be surprised if a therapist also gives you a set of hand exercises to increase your strength and range of motion (see "Exercises for the hands," page 43). He or she may also order a custom-made splint to provide rest or support for a particular part of the hand (see "Splints," page 25).

Beyond relieving immediate pain, hand therapists can help you prevent future damage to your hands by showing you how to use ergonomic tools that relieve stress on your hands, and how to set up your work space and position your body to protect your joints. They can also show you how to modify your movements and pace your activity to speed recovery.

To find a hand therapist, contact the Hand Therapy Certification Commission (see "Resources," page 50). Note that insurance coverage of hand therapy services varies; check your plan for details.

(with fingers on one side of an object and thumb on the other, as when holding a pencil); and lateral pinch (with thumb against the side of the index finger, as when holding and using a key). Grip strength is used as an indicator of health in the elderly, with a weaker grip strength one sign of frailty.

Professionals who treat hand problems

Your primary care provider or internist can diagnose and treat certain hand conditions. But in many cases, he or she may refer you to a doctor such as a rheumatologist, who specializes in arthritis and related conditions, or a general orthopedist, who specializes in muscle, tendon, bone, and joint disorders. Orthopedists are also trained in treating the forearms, elbows, and shoulders (known collectively as the upper extremities).

Hand surgeons are orthopedic, plastic, or general surgeons who have additional training in surgery of the hand. They diagnose and treat problems of the hands, wrists, and upper extremities using both surgical and nonsurgical techniques.

Occupational and physical therapists also treat hand problems. People with hand conditions may be referred to a hand therapist before seeing other physician specialists. Hand therapists teach exercises, help with proper body movement and posture, and give advice on ergonomics, with the goal of increasing strength and mobility and preventing recurring injuries. These specialists also recommend treatments, splints, and devices that make it easier to carry out the tasks of daily living, both at home and at work. A certified hand therapist is an occupational or physical therapist with at least five years of experience who specializes in rehabilitating people with hand conditions and passes a national exam on hand therapy (see "How a certified hand therapist can help," page 4). Some even specialize in treating people from particular professions. In this report, the term "therapist" refers to any of these professionals.

▶ Did you know?

About 10% of people are left-handed. Perhaps because they're in the minority, the Latin word for left, sinister, also came to mean unlucky or inauspicious. Popular notions abounded that lefties were more prone to accidents or illnesses. Studies have failed to uphold those assertions. However, living left-handed in a right-handed world can be awkward. Items as common as scissors, clothing clasps, and door handles—all designed for righties—conspire to make everyday life difficult. That said, the ranks of high achievers are filled with notable lefties, including Bill Gates, Babe Ruth, and five of the past eight U.S. presidents.

Arthritis of the hand

Joint inflammation, or arthritis, is the leading cause of disability among Americans, causing stiffness, swelling, pain, and loss of motion and function. There are more than 100 kinds of arthritis, including osteoarthritis and rheumatoid arthritis. Arthritis can affect any joint in the body, but it is most visible when it affects the hands.

Osteoarthritis

The most common of all joint diseases, osteoarthritis affects cartilage, the resilient tissue that cushions the ends of your bones. Normally, cartilage provides a smooth, gliding surface so the joints can move easily. In osteoarthritis, the cartilage thins and loses its elasticity. As the cartilage breaks down, the underlying bone may form a bony growth called a spur, or osteophyte. Fluid-filled cysts may form in the bone near the joint (see "Finger cysts," page 7). The synovial membrane lining the joints becomes inflamed, triggering the release of proteins that may damage the cartilage further.

More than 30 million Americans have osteoarthritis. In addition to the hands, osteoarthritis most commonly strikes the knees, hips, feet, and spine. The incidence rises with age, with most cases occurring in people older than 50. Heredity seems to play a role in a person's susceptibility to arthritis, particularly for osteoarthritis in the hands. Muscle weakness and a history of joint injuries caused by sports or accidents may also make a person more prone to a type of osteoarthritis known as traumatic arthritis. Ordinary, repetitive activities such as typing or playing a musical instrument may worsen arthritis symptoms, but they do not cause osteoarthritis of the hands.

There are more than 100 types of arthritis. A number of them—including osteoarthritis, rheumatoid arthritis, gout, and pseudogout—can affect the hands.

Diagnosing osteoarthritis

To diagnose any type of arthritis, your doctor may order blood tests to rule out other possible causes of your symptoms. He or she will ask specific questions about your symptoms, such as when they first started and how they affect your life. Details of your personal and family medical history may also be relevant.

Your doctor will take x-rays of the affected joints, which can reveal evidence of bone spurs and signs of cartilage breakdown within the joint. Most people older than 60 have signs of arthritis on an x-ray, but only about one-third have symptoms. There is often a big difference between the severity of osteoarthritis seen on an x-ray and how much pain and disability a person feels.

Certain joints of the hands are especially susceptible to osteoarthritis:
- **The distal interphalangeal (DIP) joint**—the last joint before the nail on each finger (see Figure 1, page 3)—is the most common site for osteoarthritis of the hands. These joints sometimes develop fibrous, bony nodules called Heberden's nodes.

> ▶ **Symptoms of osteoarthritis**
> ✔ Pain in the morning, which gradually recedes but returns at the end of the day
> ✔ Pain that is alleviated by resting the affected joint
> ✔ Stiffness in the affected joint

▶ Finger cysts

Mucous cysts are clear or flesh-colored nodules that form on the fingers under the skin at the DIP joints. They occur most commonly in middle-aged or older women with osteoarthritis. These cysts often don't cause any symptoms, but sometimes are tender and painful and may limit your finger mobility, leading to stiffness and deformity. They rarely go away on their own and may drain spontaneously and become infected, requiring prolonged antibiotic treatment. More stubborn cysts may require a hand surgeon, who will open the joint and remove the cyst as well as any associated bone growth or spur (osteophyte).

- **The basal or first carpometacarpal (CMC) joint**—located at the base of the thumb, where the thumb and wrist come together—is the second most common joint to develop osteoarthritis of the hands. Past injuries to this joint, such as a fracture or sprain, may increase the odds of getting arthritis in this joint.
- **The proximal interphalangeal (PIP) joint**—the middle joint of each finger—can also develop osteoarthritis, causing the fingers to stiffen and swell. Fibrous and bony nodules, known as Bouchard's nodes, may develop in these joints.
- **The metacarpophalangeal (MCP) joints**—where the fingers join the rest of the hand—are sometimes affected by osteoarthritis as well. These knuckle joints act as hinges between the long bones in the hand and the smaller bones in the fingers. Swelling of these joints, which may give the hands a spindle-like appearance, is common in people with rheumatoid arthritis. Injuries or other diseases, such as gout or psoriasis, can also cause problems in these joints.

Treating arthritic hands

Managing pain and improving function are the key goals in treating osteoarthritis. The best approach is usually a combination of different therapies, which can include splinting, joint protection, heat or cold therapy, exercise, medication, alternative remedies, and, in some cases, surgery.

Splinting. The first line of action for treating arthritis hand pain is splinting to immobilize the joint. This allows the joint to rest so the initial pain can subside. Splints can be used to support the painful joint during the day or at night.

Joint protection. If you have osteoarthritis, it's important to learn to recognize your body's signals to stop or slow down. A hand therapist can help you with this. To prevent pain caused by overexertion, take time to rest, and pace yourself by taking frequent breaks. Using specialized ergonomic tools and assistive devices can also make a big difference (see "Getting a grip: Handy gadgets and advice," page 47). Modifying tasks to make them less stressful allows you to continue to do the things you need or want to do while alleviating the symptoms of arthritis.

Heat or cold therapy. You can often soothe painful joints without medications. Running your hands under warm water can ease pain and stiffness and make it easier to do recommended hand exercises. Other times, usually after exercise or exertion, cold therapy may work better. You can place a bag of ice or frozen vegetables wrapped in a towel on the joint or use a freezer gel pack, available at drugstores. Check with a doctor or therapist to find out whether heat or cold is the best treatment for you.

Does knuckle cracking cause arthritis?

Cracking your knuckles may provoke an annoyed grimace from those around you, but it probably won't raise your risk for arthritis. That's the conclusion of several studies that compared rates of hand arthritis among habitual knuckle-crackers and people who didn't crack their knuckles.

The "pop" of a cracked knuckle is caused by bubbles bursting in the synovial fluid. The bubbles pop when you pull the bones apart, either by stretching the fingers or bending them backward, creating negative pressure. One study's authors compared the sudden, vibratory energy produced during knuckle cracking to "the forces responsible for the destruction of hydraulic blades and ship propellers."

Even if knuckle cracking doesn't cause arthritis, there's still good reason to let go of the habit. Chronic knuckle-crackers were more likely to have swollen hands and reduced grip strength. And there are at least two published reports of injuries suffered while people were trying to crack their knuckles.

Table 1: Topical pain relievers

Topical pain relievers work best on joints close to the skin surface, such as those in the hands. One of these, diclofenac, is only available by prescription as either a gel or patch; both forms relieve mild to moderate joint pain and inflammation. The others, which are available over the counter, are moderately effective for mild pain. None, however, will alter the course of arthritis. Do not use these on broken or irritated skin or in combination with a heating pad or bandage.

GENERIC NAME (BRAND NAME)	ACTIVE INGREDIENT	HOW IT WORKS	SIDE EFFECTS	COMMENTS
capsaicin (Capzasin, Zostrix, others)	Derived from cayenne peppers	Depletes substance P, which is believed to send pain messages to the brain	Temporary burning or stinging at the application site, which usually disappears within a few weeks of continuous use	Wash your hands thoroughly after use. Avoid contact with the eyes.
counterirritants (ArthriCare, Eucalyptamint, Icy Hot, Therapeutic Mineral Ice, others)	Include pungent oils derived from mint, wintergreen, eucalyptus, and other plants	Stimulate or irritate nerve endings to distract the brain's awareness of pain	Skin redness and irritation at application site	Many of these products have strong odors.
diclofenac (Voltaren Gel, Flector Patch)	A nonsteroidal anti-inflammatory drug (NSAID)	Inhibits hormone-like substances (prostaglandins) that contribute to pain and inflammation		Do not use with oral NSAIDs. Long-term users of either product should receive periodic blood tests to monitor liver function. All NSAIDs slightly increase the risk of heart attack and stroke, but levels that reach the bloodstream are far lower with topical application.
salicylates (Aspercreme, Bengay, Flexall, Mobisyl, Sportscreme, others)	A type of NSAID derived from willow tree bark	Same as for both diclofenac and counterirritants (see above)		Do not use if you are allergic to aspirin or are taking blood thinners.

Exercise. Exercise helps people with osteoarthritis in many ways: by improving mood, decreasing pain, and increasing flexibility and fitness over all. Therapeutic exercises, especially range-of-motion exercises for the thumb and wrist, help keep hand joints working as well as possible (see "Exercises for the hands," page 43). Gentle, pain-free strengthening may be appropriate once localized swelling and pain have subsided. Activities to improve dexterity may help counter weakness in small muscles of the hands. Consult a hand therapist for specific exercises for your hand problem, since doing the wrong type of exercise for your particular condition may make the problem worse.

Medication. There are a number of medications for arthritis, starting with topical pain relievers (see Table 1, above). One prescription gel, diclofenac (Voltaren), offers modest relief for hand arthritis. Other over-the-counter gels and creams haven't been studied as thoroughly, but some people find them helpful in treating mild to moderate pain. Topical medications can be a good choice for people with gastrointestinal conditions, since they're absorbed directly through the skin.

For more severe pain, oral medications are typically more effective (see Table 2, page 9). Those that are in the class known as nonsteroidal anti-inflammatory drugs (NSAIDs), such as the over-the-counter pain relievers ibuprofen (Advil, Motrin) and naproxen (Aleve), also curb inflammation. A drug used for rheumatoid arthritis, hydroxychloroquine (Plaquenil; see Table 3, page 11), was tested but found to be ineffective in reducing symptoms of hand osteoarthritis.

For short-term relief, corticosteroids, known informally as steroids, can be injected directly into a joint to relieve pain. Be aware, however, that excessive injections actually increase the destruction of bone and cartilage.

Table 2: Over-the-counter oral pain relievers

All of these medications except acetaminophen are NSAIDs. Avoid NSAIDs if you have gastrointestinal problems, and take them with food, milk, or an antacid to minimize stomach problems. NSAIDs other than aspirin slightly increase the risk of heart attacks and strokes.

GENERIC NAME (BRAND NAME)	USE	SIDE EFFECTS	COMMENTS
acetaminophen (Tylenol, others)	Relieves pain	Nausea, vomiting, diarrhea, jaundice, rash, tiredness, weakness; less likely to cause gastric bleeding than other pain relievers	Drinking large amounts of alcohol during long-term therapy with acetaminophen may cause liver damage. Kidney damage also possible with long-term use.
aspirin (Bayer, Bufferin, others)	Reduces inflammation and relieves pain	Stomach pain, bleeding, ulcers	High doses may cause ringing in the ears. Before using, let your doctor know if you are on blood thinners or have liver or kidney problems.
ibuprofen* (Advil, Motrin, others)			Stronger and generally longer-lasting than aspirin.
naproxen* (Aleve)			Longer-lasting than ibuprofen. .

*Ibuprofen and naproxen are available in higher doses by prescription only. Naproxen is also sold by prescription in combination with a medication to suppress stomach acid (either lansoprazole or esomeprazole), under the brand names Prevacid NapraPAC 500 and Vimovo.

Alternative or complementary therapies. These span a wide range of treatments, including yoga, acupuncture, and dietary supplements. (See "Alternative and complementary treatments for arthritis," page 13, for details.)

Surgery. This option usually is recommended only after other treatments have failed. Several surgical procedures are used for osteoarthritis, the most common being the removal of cysts and osteophytes at the DIP joint. People with severe osteoarthritis may be candidates for joint fusion or joint replacement (see the Special Section, page 17).

Rheumatoid arthritis

Rheumatoid arthritis is much less common than osteoarthritis. Still, it affects about more than 1.3 million Americans, about 70% of them women. Certain genes may make people more likely to have the disease, which can run in families.

A chronic inflammatory condition, rheumatoid arthritis most commonly strikes the small joints of the wrist, hands, and feet. However, it can also attack the joints in the neck, shoulders, elbows, hips, knees, and ankles. Misshapen fingers that make many everyday tasks nearly impossible are one telltale sign of advanced disease. Rheumatoid arthritis usually affects both sides of the body in a symmetrical fashion. Affected joints often swell, feel warm and tender, and are especially stiff and painful when you wake up or after you rest.

The disease is widely considered to be an autoimmune disorder, meaning the body's immune system goes awry and mistakenly attacks its own organs or tissues. In rheumatoid arthritis, the immune system attacks the synovium (joint lining), which then releases enzymes that destroy nearby cartilage. This causes redness, pain, and swelling. Eventually, the joints become enlarged, which hinders normal movement. Your fingers may swell and appear sausage-shaped, and you may develop a soft, lumpy mass over the back of your hand. You may hear a creaking sound (called crepitus) when you move your fingers.

Over time, the ligaments and tendons that hold bones in place stretch and weaken, causing your bones

▶ Symptoms of rheumatoid arthritis

- ✔ Swelling, warmth, and stiffness in the affected joints, especially in the morning or after rest
- ✔ Usually affects joints on both sides of the body
- ✔ In some cases, also fatigue, loss of appetite and energy, fever, or anemia

to become misaligned. The MCP joints are often affected. Your fingers may shift away from the thumb, a problem known as ulnar deviation or ulnar drift. The pain and deformity can be quite debilitating. You may find it hard to hold a cup, tool, or eating utensil. Other daily tasks such as combing your hair and buttoning your shirt can be challenging. (See "Getting a grip: Handy gadgets and advice," page 47, for tips on coping with these limitations.)

Inflammation from rheumatoid arthritis can cause the tendons to swell and rupture, resulting in an inability to extend or flex the fingers. These tendon injuries can create characteristic deformities. One condition of this type is called a boutonniere deformity, from the French word for buttonhole, so named because it involves a small tendon tear that resembles a buttonhole. Another is a swan-neck deformity, in which the middle joint of the finger (the PIP joint) hyperextends (see Figure 2, below left, and Figure 3, below).

Diagnosing rheumatoid arthritis

In addition to a medical history and physical exam, doctors use both imaging and lab tests to diagnose rheumatoid arthritis. No single lab test can confirm whether a person has rheumatoid arthritis, but several blood tests can help clarify the diagnosis. For example, about 80% of people with rheumatoid arthritis have an antibody known as rheumatoid factor in their blood, although they may not have it early on. Another blood test is for C-reactive protein (CRP), which is a sign of inflammation. X-rays can reveal swelling of soft tissues, bone loss around the joints, and bone damage (called erosions) near the joints. More sophisticated imaging tests such as magnetic resonance imaging

Figure 2: Two common finger problems from rheumatoid arthritis

When inflammation damages tendons and ligaments that normally keep a joint straight, the fingers can become deformed.

Boutonniere deformity results from damage to tendons that straighten the middle joint of the finger.

Swan-neck deformity occurs when inflammation stretches ligaments that keep fingers in proper alignment.

Figure 3: Hands with rheumatoid arthritis in many joints

These photos and x-rays come from two patients and show some of the many hand problems that can occur in rheumatoid arthritis. The pointers highlight just a few of them.

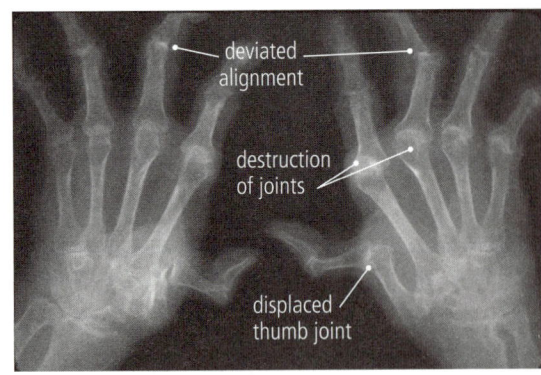

Images reprinted with permission, Barry P. Simmons, M.D.

Table 3: Medications for inflammatory arthritis

These medications are prescribed for people with rheumatoid arthritis and related types of inflammatory arthritis, such as psoriatic arthritis.

GENERIC NAME (BRAND NAME)	SIDE EFFECTS/COMMENTS
Disease-modifying antirheumatic drugs (DMARDs) These powerful drugs are prescribed early to relieve pain and swelling, limit joint damage, and alter the course of the disease.	
hydroxychloroquine (Plaquenil) leflunomide (Arava) methotrexate (Folex, Rheumatrex, Trexall) sulfasalazine (Azulfidine)	Can take weeks or months to work. Side effects vary with each medication and include increased risk for infection, hair loss, stomach upset, rash, and kidney or liver damage. Any of these drugs may interact with other medications. Methotrexate can suppress the immune system and may cause birth defects. Leflunomide may also cause birth defects. All DMARDs require close supervision and monitoring by a physician.
Kinase inhibitor This one-of-a-kind drug affects the inflammatory mechanism inside cells and is used for moderate to severe rheumatoid arthritis in people who do not respond to methotrexate or another DMARD.	
tofacitinib (Xeljanz)	Pill taken twice daily. Reduces inflammation. Side effects may include diarrhea, headache, runny or stuffy nose, and sore throat.
Biological response modifiers These drugs, also known as biologics, are created from genetically engineered proteins derived from human genes. Given by injection or intravenous infusion, they inhibit specific components of the immune system, helping to suppress inflammation and slow the progression of rheumatoid arthritis.	
Anti-TNF compounds: • adalimumab (Humira) • certolizumab (Cimzia) • etanercept (Enbrel) • golimumab (Simponi) • infliximab (Remicade)	Side effects vary depending on the medication and include an increased risk for infections, from colds and sinus infections to more serious diseases such as tuberculosis.
Other biological response modifiers: • abatacept (Orencia) • anakinra (Kineret) • rituximab (Rituxan) • sarilumab (Kevzara) • secukinumab (Cosentix) • tocilizumab (Actemra)	Side effects vary but may include nausea, diarrhea, heartburn, muscle or back pain, tiredness, weakness, numbness in the hands or feet, stomach area pain. Tocilizumab may cause serious infections, diverticulitis, severe allergic reactions, and increases in blood lipids.

(MRI) can detect early inflammation, even before it's visible on an x-ray, and can pinpoint synovitis (inflammation of the lining of the joint).

Treating rheumatoid arthritis

As with osteoarthritis, doctors recommend painkillers (see Table 1, page 8, and Table 2, page 9), and, in some cases, corticosteroids to help manage pain and swelling. But decades of research show that early treatment with powerful drugs known as disease-modifying antirheumatic drugs (DMARDs) can lessen the chance of long-term disability from rheumatoid arthritis for some people. As a result, most people with rheumatoid arthritis take a DMARD, usually methotrexate. Another option is a group of drugs known as biological response modifiers, which work by inhibiting specific components of the immune system (see Table 3, above, for more details).

Because DMARDs have proven so successful in keeping rheumatoid arthritis at bay and reducing joint destruction, hand surgeons have seen a decline in the number of people who need surgery. But for those whose symptoms become debilitating despite medical therapies, surgery is an option. Surgery for rheumatoid arthritis strives to reduce pain and improve function, and can also improve the appearance of your hands.

Soft tissue removal (particularly procedures known as synovectomy and tenosynovectomy) involves removing diseased tissue from the tendons and joints. The surgeon may also reposition some tendons and release others to stop the fingers from drifting toward the little finger. Although synovectomy can decrease pain and swelling and slow joint destruction, the condition may recur. However, use of DMARDs dramatically decreases recurrence.

In rare instances, surgeons replace wrist joints (and in some cases, MCP and PIP joints) destroyed by rheumatoid arthritis (see the Special Section, "Joint reconstruction for arthritic hands," page 17).

Physical or occupational therapy for rheumatoid arthritis of the hands is similar to treatment for osteoarthritis and includes splinting, joint protection, pacing, ergonomics, and gentle exercise. These therapies may be key to managing your symptoms and regaining your function. It's important to seek medical advice early because it may help you detect when the condition is getting worse and begin treatment to prevent deformities.

Other types of arthritis that affect the hands

Several other, less-common types of arthritis, including gout and pseudogout, can cause debilitating hand symptoms. In addition, conditions such as lupus, scleroderma, and psoriatic arthritis may cause arthritic symptoms that involve the hands.

Gout

Gout accounts for about 5% of all cases of arthritis. This condition is caused by deposits of tiny, needle-like crystals that form when the body either makes too much uric acid or excretes too little of it. Uric acid forms from the breakdown of purine, a substance found in protein-rich foods. The symptoms of gout resemble those of rheumatoid arthritis (joint pain, tenderness, warmth, and redness), but gout tends to affect only one joint at a time, and it may begin suddenly—often in the middle of the night. Pain may be quite severe and tends to resolve within a few days. Gout is most common in the big toe joint (a condition known as podagra). However, it often affects other joints in the feet, ankles, and hands, as well as elsewhere in the body.

> **Symptoms of gout**
> ✔ Jolts of pain in the affected joint
> ✔ Possible inflammation of the joint
> ✔ Increase in symptoms after eating certain foods

Anyone can get gout, but it's most common in men older than 40. In women, it is most likely to develop after menopause. Gout occurs in about one in 100 people over all, but in as many as 6% to 7% of older men. Being overweight and drinking excessive amounts of alcohol increase your risk for gout. Research suggests that men who eat generous amounts of red meat and seafood are more prone to gout. Those who eat more low-fat dairy products are less likely to be affected.

To diagnose gout, doctors measure uric acid levels in the blood and take a sample of fluid from the joint to look for uric acid crystals under a special microscope. But uric acid levels aren't always elevated during an attack, and many people with high levels never develop gout. Some people develop lumpy deposits made of sodium urate (called tophi) around the joints.

Treatment usually involves NSAIDs (see Table 2, page 9), but not aspirin, which can raise uric acid levels. People who can't take NSAIDs or who aren't helped by them may take a corticosteroid, either in pill form or by injection.

Some people with gout are prescribed drugs to lower uric acid levels in their blood. These include probenecid (Benemid, Probalan) to increase urinary excretion of uric acid, and allopurinol (Zyloprim), febuxostat (Uloric), and pegloticase (Krystexxa) to reduce the body's production of uric acid. Lesinurad (Zurampic), which has a different mechanism for increasing uric acid excretion, is used in combination with allopurinol or febuxostat.

Alternative and complementary treatments for arthritis

Many people with chronic, painful conditions like arthritis who don't get complete relief from conventional therapies turn to alternative treatments. As with any therapy, some people find that certain treatments work well for them, while others find little or no benefit. Talk with your physician to decide which approaches might work best for you, and consult a licensed, certified practitioner for specific treatment and guidance. *The discussion below does not constitute an endorsement of any of these treatments.*

Yoga. A 2011 review of 11 studies of yoga for treating arthritis suggests that yoga helps ease symptoms such as tender, swollen joints; pain; and disability. Several types of yoga classes are available in most communities; be sure to choose one with a gentle style, ideally taught by an instructor familiar with hand problems and the therapeutic uses of yoga.

Acupuncture and acupressure. These ancient Chinese therapies have become popular for treating pain-related conditions, and some studies have shown acupuncture to be effective for some forms of pain. A 2013 analysis also indicates that the therapy can be useful in the treatment of gout. However, there are no specific studies demonstrating the effectiveness of acupuncture for treating hand pain.

Diet. Several studies indicate that there is a connection between diet and the systemic inflammation that characterizes rheumatoid arthritis. A diet emphasizing fruits and vegetables, olive oil, fish, and whole grains—similar to the Mediterranean eating pattern—may reduce inflammation.

Dietary supplements. A number of vitamins, minerals, and other substances are sold as remedies for arthritis. Because these products are classified as dietary supplements, they are not scrutinized for effectiveness and purity by the FDA. The following supplements have been tested for various forms of arthritis within the past decade:

- **Avocado soybean unsaponifiables.** In a meta-analysis of four studies using a proprietary combination product, there was moderate-quality evidence that the supplement slightly improved pain and function.
- **Boswellia serrate (Indian frankincense).** In a meta-analysis combining two studies, patients who took the supplement for 90 days reported slightly less pain and increased function compared with individuals who took a placebo.
- **Curcumin (turmeric).** In a monthlong trial, curcumin supplements were as effective as ibuprofen in treating knee osteoarthritis, with fewer gastrointestinal side effects.
- **Glucosamine and chondroitin sulfate.** Although limited research has been conducted on glucosamine and chondroitin sulfate for osteoarthritis of the hand, a small trial done in 2011 showed that the supplements may have promise. The people who used the treatment reported less pain and morning stiffness and increased hand function over the individuals in the control group. Recent studies in patients with arthritis in other joints have had conflicting results.
- **Omega-3 fatty acids.** Some evidence suggests these fatty acids, found in fish oil, help curb inflammation in rheumatoid arthritis. Mild side effects include belching, bad breath, and other minor gastrointestinal problems.

Pseudogout

As its name suggests, pseudogout is similar to gout, except that the crystals in the joints are made of calcium pyrophosphate dihydrate. The condition is often referred to as calcium pyrophosphate deposition disease, abbreviated as CPDD. Like gout, pseudogout causes redness, heat, and swelling in one or more joints, including those in the wrists and knees. The body attacks the crystals, which can cause swelling that may damage nearby cartilage.

About 3% of people in their 60s develop pseudogout, although not all of them will have attacks. No

▶ Symptoms of pseudogout

✔ Jolts of pain in the affected joint
✔ Redness, warmth, and swelling in the affected joint

one knows why some people develop these crystals, but they may result from an abnormality in the cartilage cells or connective tissue. Genes may also have an influence, and people with certain other medical conditions, including hypercalcemia (excessive calcium in the blood), hypothyroidism (low activity of the thyroid gland), and hemochromatosis (excess iron in the blood), are more prone to the problem.

Samples of joint fluid can help doctors diagnose pseudogout, and x-rays may reveal the calcium deposits in the joint. Drug treatments for a sudden attack of pseudogout are the same as those for gout: NSAIDs and corticosteroids. Sometimes removing joint fluid by needle aspiration improves the condition without additional treatment.

Lupus

An autoimmune disease related to rheumatoid arthritis, lupus can affect various parts of the body, especially the skin, blood, and kidneys, as well as the joints—including multiple joints in the hand and wrist. Also called systemic lupus erythematosus (SLE), the disease affects women about eight to 10 times as often as men, most commonly between the ages of 18 and 45. Lupus-related arthritis in the hands tends to cause less swelling and actual joint damage than rheumatoid arthritis, but it may affect similar joints and feel the same.

Some people with lupus develop hand deformities similar to those seen in rheumatoid arthritis, such as ulnar deviation and swan-neck deformities (see Figure 3, page 10). It can be hard to diagnose because there isn't a specific set of symptoms that occurs in everyone with the disease. The workup may include several different blood tests, as well as urine analysis, chest x-rays, and heart tests. Medical treatments for lupus include painkillers (see Table 2, page 9) as well as some drugs used to treat rheumatoid arthritis, such as methotrexate and hydroxychloroquine, an antimalaria drug (see Table 3, page 11).

Symptoms of lupus
- ✔ Swollen, achy joints
- ✔ Fever (100° F or higher)
- ✔ Prolonged or extreme fatigue
- ✔ Rashes

Symptoms of scleroderma
- ✔ Hard, thickened skin that appears shiny and may lose hair
- ✔ Swollen, puffy fingers and toes with poor blood flow and extreme sensitivity to cold
- ✔ Ulcers or sores on fingers
- ✔ In some cases, digestive, heart, lung, or kidney problems

Scleroderma

This autoimmune, rheumatic disease commonly affects the hands and fingers. Derived from the Greek words meaning "hard skin," scleroderma is also a connective tissue disease, meaning it affects major substances in the skin, tendons, and bones. It can be either localized (affecting limited areas of the skin, muscles, and bones) or systemic (causing more widespread skin changes and sometimes damaging the lungs, heart, and kidneys). It is quite rare, with only 10 to 20 new cases diagnosed per million people each year, mostly in women.

People with scleroderma often have some or all of the symptoms that doctors refer to as CREST, which stands for the following:

- **Calcinosis:** the formation of calcium deposits (visible on x-rays) in connective tissues, usually in the fingertips, face, and trunk, and on the skin above the elbows and knees. Painful ulcers may form where the deposits break through the skin.
- **Raynaud's syndrome:** a condition that occurs when small blood vessels in the hands or feet contract in response to cold (see "Cold hands: Is it Raynaud's syndrome?" on page 15).
- **Esophageal dysfunction:** a condition caused by muscle problems in the esophagus (the tube that connects the throat and stomach), making swallowing difficult and sometimes causing chronic heartburn.
- **Sclerodactyly:** thick, tight skin on the fingers, stemming from too much connective tissue within

Continued on page 16

Cold hands: Is it Raynaud's syndrome?

If your fingers turn ghostly white and numb when exposed to cold, you may have Raynaud's syndrome. A common condition (it affects up to one in 10 people, most of them women), Raynaud's is an exaggeration of the body's normal response to cold. It usually affects the hands and feet and, less often, the nose, lips, and ears. Many people are extremely sensitive to the cold, but unless your extremities actually change color—to either white from lack of blood or blue from poorly oxygenated blood—you don't have Raynaud's.

The best treatment for Raynaud's is to avoid sudden and unprotected exposure to cold temperatures. Wear vests and gloves. Preheat your car.

When exposed to cold, the body normally slows its loss of heat and tries to preserve its core temperature. Blood vessels near the surface constrict, redirecting blood flow deeper into the body. In Raynaud's, this process is more extreme and can occur even with a fairly small decrease in air temperature.

An episode of Raynaud's begins when the blood vessels supplying the fingers and toes contract spasmodically, hampering the flow of oxygen-rich blood to the skin. Some of these vessels even collapse. The skin becomes pale and cool, sometimes blanching to a stark white color. The affected tissues may become numb and cold, and people with Raynaud's are more susceptible to frostbite than other people. However, a key feature of Raynaud's is that it is reversible. When the blood vessels finally relax and blood flow resumes, the skin becomes warm and flushed—and very red. The fingers or toes may throb or tingle.

Some people with Raynaud's have other health problems, usually connective tissue disorders such as scleroderma or lupus. Your doctor can determine this by doing a physical exam, asking you about your symptoms, and taking a few blood tests. But most of the time, there is no underlying medical problem.

The best treatment for Raynaud's is to prevent episodes, mainly by avoiding sudden and unprotected exposure to cold temperatures. Keeping your whole body warm helps prevent the reflexive constriction of blood vessels in your skin. Before you head outside into the cold, put on gloves and warm footwear, but also bundle up your entire body and head, taking advantage of items such as silk underwear, vests, and lightweight activewear. Preheat your car before getting in. You may want to wear gloves in chilly grocery store aisles and when reaching into your own freezer, if you find that action triggers the problem. Even exposure to air conditioning may be troublesome for people with Raynaud's.

It's also a good idea to avoid things that cause your blood vessels to constrict. Smoking is one such aggravating factor. Certain medications may also constrict the blood vessels; these include amphetamines, cold and allergy formulas that contain phenylephrine or pseudoephedrine, and migraine drugs that contain ergotamine. Stressful events may also provoke an episode of Raynaud's. After a large meal, blood is diverted from the extremities to the digestive system, so keep food intake moderate.

Relaxation techniques can help prevent stress-induced episodes. Thermal biofeedback, which trains people to self-regulate their finger temperature, also shows some promise in treating Raynaud's. This technique uses sensors placed on the fingers that feed temperature information to a video screen, so you can monitor your progress.

Your doctor may prescribe a medication that relaxes the blood vessels, usually a calcium-channel blocker. If it's not effective, other blood pressure drugs that open up blood vessels may help. Drugs used to treat erectile dysfunction (which work by expanding blood vessels and boosting blood flow) have been found to have a moderate effect in easing Raynaud's symptoms. You may not need to take these drugs all the time, but only during the cold season, when Raynaud's tends to be worse.

In severe cases that have not responded to other therapy, case reports indicate that injections of botulinum toxin A (Botox, Dysport, Xeomin) may improve blood flow in the fingers and reduce symptoms. Research trials are ongoing.

If medical treatment fails to provide adequate relief of symptoms, a surgical procedure called sympathectomy is an option. Surgical sympathectomy removes the small nerves that surround the blood vessels of the hands and fingers, allowing maximum dilation of these vessels.

Once a Raynaud's episode starts, it's important to get warm as quickly as possible. Try soaking your hands in lukewarm (about 105° F) water, or put them under your armpits or in another warm area. But don't put your hands, feet, or face on a heater or anything else that could scald or otherwise injure you.

Continued from page 14

skin layers. Bending or straightening the fingers becomes difficult, and the skin may become shiny, dark, and hairless. The fingertips become tapered and may ulcerate.

- **Telangiectasias**: small red spots on the hands and face caused by the swelling of tiny blood vessels, which are not painful but may be unsightly.

Doctors also rely on blood tests, and possibly skin biopsies, to confirm a diagnosis of scleroderma. But such tests aren't definitive. Scleroderma symptoms vary and may come and go, especially in milder cases, making the disease difficult to diagnose.

Because there is no cure for scleroderma, treatments are meant to relieve symptoms. For example, blood pressure drugs that help widen blood vessels can help ease Raynaud's syndrome, and acid-lowering drugs can ease heartburn symptoms. NSAIDs or other painkillers help treat muscle pain. Hand therapy for scleroderma includes stretching and range-of-motion exercises, gentle massage and splinting to reduce joint contractures, paraffin treatments to soften skin, and help with modifying routine activities to limit stress on tender joints and relieve joint pain and swelling (see "Getting a grip: Handy gadgets and advice," page 47).

Psoriatic arthritis

This uncommon type of arthritis is related to psoriasis, a chronic skin condition marked by thick, red patches of skin covered with silvery scales. About a quarter of people with psoriasis develop psoriatic arthritis. In most cases, the skin condition is diagnosed first, but the arthritis may occur before the first signs of psoriasis, and some people with the condition have no skin lesions at all. Psoriatic arthritis can strike at any age but usually occurs between the ages of 20 and 50.

The condition often affects the fingernails, causing small indentations (pitting) or lifting of the nails. As with all types of arthritis, joint swelling, stiffness, and pain are common; unlike rheumatoid arthritis, psoriatic arthritis usually affects only a few joints and tends to be asymmetric (that is, joints on both sides of the body are not necessarily affected similarly). Diagnosis is based on the person's history of psoriasis; physical examination of the skin, nails, and joints; x-rays; and, in some cases, joint fluid tests. Treatments for psoriatic arthritis include those used for rheumatoid arthritis, such as steroids, topical and oral NSAIDs, and DMARDs (see Table 1, page 8; Table 2, page 9; and Table 3, page 11). Hand therapy treatments include reducing activity, protecting the joint, controlling swelling, improving range of motion, and learning gentle stretching and strengthening techniques.

Symptoms of psoriatic arthritis

✔ Joint swelling, stiffness, and pain in one or more joints
✔ Pitting of the fingernails and toenails
✔ In some cases, silver or gray scaly spots on the scalp, elbows, knees, or lower spine

SPECIAL SECTION

Joint reconstruction for arthritic hands

Replacing knee, hip, and shoulder joints is almost routine these days. Replacing hand joints is more challenging, because of the smaller joint size and the intricate structure of both the wrist and digits. But advances in materials and mechanics have made replacing hand joints—including the entire wrist, as well as knuckle and finger joints—a viable option. The need for artificial hand joints has declined somewhat in recent years, thanks to the success of drug treatments (especially DMARDs) in keeping crippling hand arthritis at bay. But joint replacement remains an important option for many people.

Thumb surgery

The most commonly replaced hand joint is the basal or first carpometacarpal (CMC) joint, located at the base of the thumb where it meets the wrist (see Figure 1, page 3). This is usually done in people with osteoarthritis. Several different techniques are used, all of which appear to be equally effective. One popular approach involves removing an arthritic trapezium (the bone at the base of the thumb) and replacing it with a piece of tendon that's taken from the person's forearm and coiled up to provide a spacer or cushion (see Figure 4, at right, and "Barbara's story," page 18). Another option is total joint replacement, in which a prosthetic joint is used; however, long-term studies show a significant rate of failure for the artificial implants.

Wrist surgery: Total joint replacement vs. fusion

Total joint replacement (arthroplasty) involves removing damaged bone or joints and replacing

---

Figure 4: Surgery for arthritis in the thumb

One common type of surgery for arthritis in the basal or first carpometacarpal (CMC) joint of the thumb is total joint reconstruction, which involves removing the arthritic trapezium that normally forms a joint with four adjacent bones. The surgeon replaces the removed bone with a coiled-up tendon from the wrist, the flexor carpi radialis, which acts as a cushion among the remaining wrist bones.

Recovery may take several months, but the final result is the return of full joint motion and pinching and gripping strength as well as pain relief. Generally, this is a highly successful operation with few complications and excellent long-term results.

Total joint replacement using an artificial implant is usually less successful in the long run.

SPECIAL SECTION | Joint reconstruction for arthritic hands

BARBARA'S STORY: Surgery for basal joint arthritis

Barbara first noticed the pain in her left thumb while picking up a small child—a routine part of her job as a preschool teacher. The 53-year-old Massachusetts woman had been diagnosed with osteoarthritis several years earlier, but hadn't been terribly bothered by the disease until her thumb started to ache and lose strength. After several conservative measures failed to relieve the pain, she opted for basal joint reconstruction surgery (see Figure 4, page 17). This is Barbara's story:

I consulted a hand surgeon, who took x-rays. The images showed the degeneration of my thumb joint, narrowing of the joint space, and bone spurs. He recommended a short opponens splint, made of lightweight, hard plastic. It's designed to immobilize the thumb so it can rest and heal. I wore the splint at night and during the day when I wasn't using my hands. During that time, I noticed that my right thumb began hurting a bit, although not as much as the left. Apparently, that's not unusual, because you tend to use your opposite hand to compensate.

But after six weeks, the pain was still there. It was like a nagging headache, but in my thumb. I then tried a long opponens splint, which reaches all the way from the thumb to the middle of the forearm. But after another six weeks, the pain was still there.

The next step was a cortisone injection, which helped for a few weeks. But within about six to eight weeks, the pain had returned. That's when I decided to have surgery.

The day of the surgery, I received an injection in my armpit to numb my entire arm. They also gave me a mild intravenous sedative to help me relax. The entire procedure took only about 45 minutes.

Afterward, my arm felt very strange, like the way your mouth feels after you've had a shot of Novocain at the dentist. Your entire arm is also quite big and bulky, because you have to wear a large bandage and cast. They gave me a sling to support my arm, but it wasn't very comfortable, so I stopped using it after a day or two.

Right after the surgery, I took Percocet. After the first day or so, I found I could control the pain by taking Tylenol every four hours.

Getting dressed was a challenge, but I quickly found creative ways to get around those problems. After 10 days, they took off the large cast and put on a smaller, hard cast that reached just to my mid-forearm. At one point, I tried gripping a golf club to see if I could swing at all, but that didn't work too well!

Right after the cast came off, my scars were quite red, but they faded fairly quickly. I found that massaging the scar helped the area feel less sensitive. My thumb was slightly swollen, and I noticed that my first finger was a little numb for a few weeks. But other than that, my hand felt fine. Every day, the pain decreased, and my mobility increased a little more.

I saw a therapist a few times. She showed me exercises to stretch my thumb and build up my thumb and wrist muscles, which had weakened while I was in the cast. It took a long time to regain my upper-body strength, but I went to the gym regularly, even while I still had the cast. I feel that yoga classes also helped, both for strengthening my arms and easing my osteoarthritis in general.

Nine months after the surgery, I was 98% back to normal.

About seven years after the first surgery, Barbara's other thumb became increasingly painful, and she eventually had the identical surgery on her right thumb.

My recovery was a little more difficult the second time around, and it took longer to heal. I think that I may not have been as vigilant about doing my exercises, and the fact that I'm right-handed made it more challenging. I still have some discomfort, but, being older and having a little arthritis, I think that just goes with the territory. Over all, though, the surgery was successful. It cured what was bothering me, and now I can function much better and do things that I couldn't do before, like brush my teeth or grasp a plate. I have no regrets about having the procedure done, and I have recommended the surgery to several other people I know who have had similar problems.

---

them with a prosthetic joint. Prosthetic joints may include silicone, polyethylene, titanium, or pyrocarbon, a substance consisting of a tough, ceramic-like coating over graphite. Compared with those of the past, today's prosthetic designs are less likely to degrade or loosen. They also provide better range of motion and greater stability, which makes everyday tasks like writing and hair combing much easier.

People with rheumatoid arthritis are the most likely candidates for a total wrist replacement. About two-thirds of people with rheumatoid arthritis have wrist symptoms within two years of their diagnosis, and that number rises to more than 90% by 10 years (see "Do you need a new joint?" at right). People with osteoarthritis or traumatic arthritis (a form of arthritis resulting from a previous fracture or ligament injury) may also benefit from the procedure.

Wrist replacement can be done under either general or regional block anesthesia as an inpatient or outpatient procedure. The surgeon removes the first row of carpal (wrist) bones and shapes the end of the radius (the main forearm bone) to fit the prosthesis. The radial component of the prosthesis inserts into the radius, while the carpal component inserts into the remaining carpal bones. A plastic spacer fits between the two components (see Figure 5, at right).

For some people with painful, damaged wrists, however, joint fusion (arthrodesis) may be a better option than replacement. Joint fusion permanently stiffens the joint to relieve pain and correct deformities that interfere with normal function or to improve the hand's appearance. The surgeon aligns the bones in the most natural position. First performed on wrists in the early 1900s, fusion provides reliable and sustained long-term pain relief with few complications. But because the bones are fused, the joint loses its normal mobility.

A review of 38 studies, which included about 500 wrist replace-

Do you need a new joint?

When is it time for a joint replacement? Joint replacement is always an elective procedure. Although your surgeon may make you aware of the possibility of joint replacement, you must weigh the benefits and risks and come to your own decision about whether, or when, to undergo this major surgery. Although age is an important factor, the decision to have a joint replacement is based on your disability—how much pain you are in and how much your joint problems limit your activities. Joint surgery—either fusion or replacement—may be a good option if one or more of the following apply to you:

- You are unable to complete normal daily tasks without help.
- You have significant pain every day.
- Pain keeps you awake at night despite the use of medications.
- Nonsurgical approaches such as medications and splints have not relieved your pain.
- Less-complicated surgical procedures are unlikely to help.
- Pain keeps you from doing daily activities or your job.
- Pain doesn't subside when you rest.
- You are suffering severe side effects from the medications needed to control your joint symptoms.

Figure 5: Wrist replacement (arthroplasty)

In a wrist replacement, a surgeon replaces the damaged wrist joint with an artificial joint that includes several metal components. The radial component inserts into the radius bone, while the carpal component is secured into the carpal bones through one long stem and two screws. A polyethylene spacer fits between the other two components in the joint area. Flat on one side and rounded on the other, the spacer's design allows it to fit into the carpal component while it rocks on the radial component, enabling a natural wrist motion.

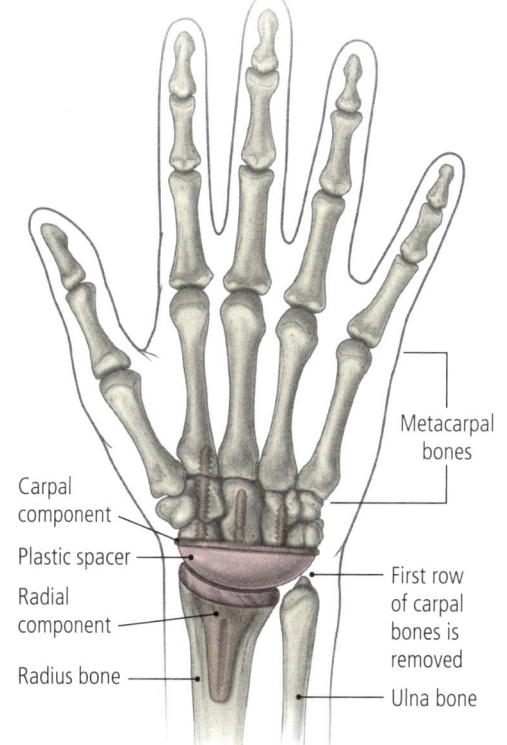

SPECIAL SECTION | Joint reconstruction for arthritic hands

ments and more than 800 wrist fusions, concluded that both procedures can relieve pain, although fusion may provide greater relief. The tradeoff, of course, is the loss of mobility. For people who need both wrists treated, experts often recommend having one wrist fused and the other replaced, which allows a broader range of function than if you have wrist fusion in both. Several studies comparing the results of people who had both treatments suggest that people prefer the results of the replacement surgery because of greater ability to move; however, replacement has historically had a higher complication rate. A failed wrist replacement—in which an implant loosens and pain and deformity occur—can be redone as a wrist fusion, but it is a challenging operation that requires bone grafting to fill the space formerly occupied by the implant.

After wrist replacement surgery, you'll first wear a plaster forearm splint, which is applied in the operating room, for about 10 days. Then a hand therapist will make a customized splint that you'll use for four to six weeks. For wrist fusion surgery, you will need to wear a splint for 10 days followed by a cast for four weeks. During your recovery, you should work with a certified hand therapist, who can help you control the pain and swelling from the surgery. She or he will demonstrate and recommend specific exercises (see "Exercises for the hands," page 43) and teach you how to grip and support items to avoid putting undue stress on your wrist. (Also see "Surgical scars," below, for tips on making your scars less noticeable.)

Surgery on finger joints

The knuckle, or MCP joint, is the joint most often affected by

Figure 6: Surgery to correct hand deformities

Before surgery

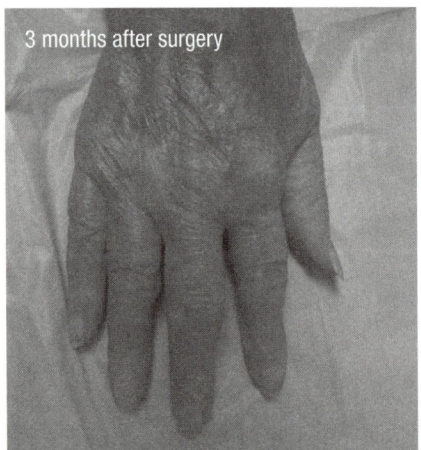
3 months after surgery

Much of the deformity caused by rheumatoid arthritis can be surgically corrected. This woman had arthroplasty of the MCP joint in her right hand plus reconstructive surgery. The surgeon removed diseased joint tissue, replaced it with silicone implants, rearranged soft tissue, and reconstructed ligaments.

Photos reprinted with permission, Barry P. Simmons, M.D.

Surgical scars

All surgeries have the potential to leave scars, but you can do things to make them less noticeable. Most surgical dressings are removed within seven to 10 days. Your scar may be red and bumpy, but it will eventually lighten and flatten. Provided the wound is completely closed and has no drainage, you can try these tips to minimize the appearance of a scar:

- Soak the area in warm water for several minutes.
- Gently massage the scar with a nonallergenic cream or lotion (such as Eucerin cream) up to five times per day. The motions should be circular, side to side, and up and down.
- Rub the scar with increasingly rough materials to help make it less sensitive. Start by rubbing it with a soft cotton cloth for a few minutes a day for a week or so. Then switch to terry cloth, and eventually to fine sandpaper.
- If your scar is raised (known as a hypertrophic scar), use a scar pad (available in drugstores), which places gentle pressure on the scar to help flatten it.
- Use sunscreen (at least SPF 15) to prevent the scar from becoming darker.
- Gentle stretching can also help, but it depends on the location of the scar.

See a therapist for recommendations for specific exercises and other advice about your particular scars.

rheumatoid arthritis of the hand, which often causes the disfiguring displacement of the fingers known as ulnar deviation, in which the fingers angle away from the thumb. These joints are condylar, meaning the bones are rounded where they form the joint. As a result, they are less stable than other finger joints, which makes replacing them especially challenging; aggressive reconstruction of the tendons and ligaments is an essential part of the procedure (see Figure 6, page 20). Surgeons have used silicone and silastic (a blend of silicone and plastic) spacers to replace damaged MCP joints. Long-term follow-up shows some deterioration of the reconstructed joints, but very few people require additional surgery to correct this. Pyrocarbon MCP joints initially appeared promising for osteoarthritis and some cases of rheumatoid arthritis, but longer follow-up has revealed complications, causing surgeons to limit their use.

As with MCP joints, surgeons have used both silicone and pyrocarbon to replace the PIP, or middle, joint of the finger. One study in the *Journal of Hand Surgery* found the two types of implants performed equally well to relieve pain and improve range of motion. The recovery from these surgeries is similar to that for a wrist joint replacement.

A pyrocarbon PIP joint replacement was approved by the FDA in 2002 as a Humanitarian Use Device. Such approvals are granted for conditions or diseases that typically affect fewer than 4,000 people in the United States per year. Early studies revealed a failure rate of 30% for the pyrocarbon implants, which dampened initial enthusiasm for them. A 2015 study in the *Journal of Hand Surgery* documented 36 additional surgeries among 97 pyrocarbon PIP joint replacements in 72 people who were followed between five and 14 years—a higher rate of additional surgeries than with other prostheses. For this reason, your surgeon may recommend a silicone implant or joint fusion instead (see Figure 7, above).

Fusion of the PIP joint is an accepted and frequently suggested procedure. Fusion has a low complication rate and a high success rate with complete relief of pain.

For the DIP joint, fusion is realistically the only procedure. It has a low complication rate and high success rate.

Preparing for hand surgery

Recovering from any surgery is hard, but making do with just one hand for several weeks (or longer)

Figure 7: Finger joint repair: Fusion vs. replacement

The x-ray on the left shows the hand of a 61-year-old woman with osteoarthritis who had joint fusion in her index-finger PIP joint and small-finger DIP joint, which required bone grafts and pins and wires to hold the joints in place.

The x-ray on the right shows an example of two PIP joint replacements, done on a 57-year-old woman with osteoarthritis. The artificial pyrocarbon joints used in this procedure (see inset) allow the fingers to bend.

Whether fusion or replacement is better for you depends on your individual case. Joint fusions have a high success rate and provide a pain-free, stable, but unmovable joint. Joint replacements allow movement and provide good pain relief, but are less reliable, meaning a repeat procedure may be needed.

X-rays reprinted with permission, Barry P. Simmons, M.D. Inset photo courtesy of Integra LifeSciences.

SPECIAL SECTION | Joint reconstruction for arthritic hands

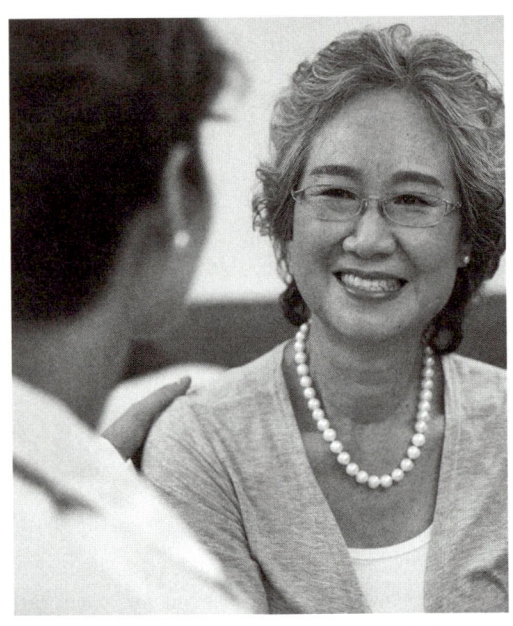

Preparing in advance for hand surgery will help your recovery go more smoothly. Fix meals that you can freeze and save; set aside loose clothes to wear.

poses some additional challenges. Taking time to prepare in advance can ease some of the inconvenience. Also, remember to pace yourself after surgery and don't overuse your other hand, which can strain or injure your hand or arm.

Get organized. Contact your insurance company in advance about coverage for the surgical procedure, follow-up office visits, and therapy visits. Make a folder to organize your bills, appointment reminders, and postoperative recommendations. Ask your doctor for an estimated recovery time, so you can talk to your employer about when you'll be able to return to work. Set up automatic bill payments, or pay bills ahead of time.

Ask for help. Enlist help in advance from family, friends, or neighbors. Get a small calendar to keep track of who will be available when. Update their phone and email addresses and keep them handy. You may need assistance with transportation to and from surgery and follow-up appointments; caring for children, pets, and plants; and doing yard work and housecleaning. Consider hiring a cleaning service, even for just one or two visits.

Modify your self-care. Practice dressing and undressing, using the bathroom, showering, and brushing and flossing your teeth with one hand. Useful tools include shampoo and toothpaste in flip-top or pump dispensers, pre-strung dental flossers, and an electric toothbrush. Keep a hairbrush in the shower to assist with shampooing. Buy a terry cloth robe for drying yourself after bathing or showering. You may need to keep your hand dry and wrap it after surgery, so check your drugstore for cast protectors.

Eat efficiently. Prepare meals ahead and freeze them. Buy frozen, microwaveable dinners. Plan for "no cut" meals such as sandwiches, ground meat, and finger foods. Make a contact list of favorite take-out and delivery options. Stock up on nonperishables.

Simplify your wardrobe. Loose clothing and clothes with large buttons—but no zippers—will ease the task of getting dressed. Slip-on shoes are a good idea, too.

Tendon trouble

Think of the tendons in your arms and hands as the strings of a marionette, enabling you to lift your wrist and hand and to move your thumb and fingers. For a variety of reasons or for no apparent reason, the tendons or tendon sheaths can become inflamed, causing pain whenever you put any tension on the tendon. Certain tendons and tendon sheaths in the fingers, wrists, and elbows are particularly prone to inflammation, leading to specific types of tendinitis, tenosynovitis, and epicondylitis.

De Quervain's tendinitis

Tendinitis is swelling of the tendon. In the wrist, the most common location for tendinitis is on the thumb side. When it occurs there, it is called de Quervain's tendinitis (also known as tenosynovitis). De Quervain's results from repetitive hand and wrist movements—for example, while gardening or playing sports. It is sometimes called "new mother's disease" because it often develops in women with newborn babies, possibly in response to the repetitive movements made while caring for an infant. The condition is far less common in new fathers.

The main symptom is pain over the thumb side of the wrist, which can appear gradually or suddenly and may move up the forearm. The pain worsens when you grasp things or twist your wrist. Picking up a coffee mug may become impossible. You may notice swelling over the affected tendon, and a fluid-filled cyst may arise in the same area. The thumb may occasionally "catch" or "snap" when you move it.

To diagnose de Quervain's, the doctor will ask you to make a fist with your fingers over the thumb and bend your wrist toward the little finger. This maneuver, known as the Finkelstein test, is usually quite painful for a person with de Quervain's. But tenderness over the tendons on the thumb side of the wrist is the most common finding.

Treatments include resting the thumb and wrist by wearing a splint (see "Splints," page 25). Your doctor may also recommend anti-inflammatory medicines to curb pain and reduce swelling. Steroid injections into the tendon compartment may help. If all these measures fail to improve your symptoms, surgery (which releases the tendon sheath) is often successful. A hand therapist can design an exercise program to restore flexibility and strength once the initial symptoms clear up.

Trigger finger

The term trigger finger may conjure up visions of sharpshooters and hunters. Actually, this condition (officially known as stenosing tenosynovitis) is most

Figure 8: Trigger finger

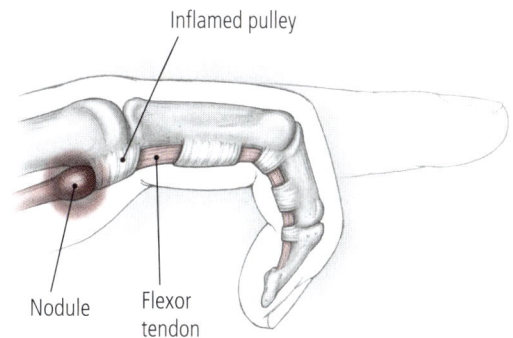

An often-painful condition, trigger finger is caused by a narrowing of the sheath that surrounds the tendon and irritation of the pulley, the ring of connective tissue that holds the tendon close to the bone. Trigger finger is most common in people over age 40 who also have rheumatoid arthritis. Symptoms include a sensation of "catching" when trying to bend or straighten the finger. A bump (nodule) may also form.

> **Symptoms of de Quervain's tendinitis**
> ✔ Pain on the thumb side of the wrist, especially when pinching, grasping, or making a fist
> ✔ A small knot or tenderness on the thumb side of the wrist

common in the ring finger and the thumb. It is called trigger finger because of the trigger-like snap that occurs when the finger briefly locks and then suddenly releases when you try to bend or straighten it. The condition affects the tendons that bend the fingers and the pulleys (rings of connective tissue) that hold those tendons close to the finger bones (see Figure 8, page 23). If the tendon develops a knot (nodule) or if the lining covering the tendon swells, it has to squeeze through the opening of the tunnel, causing pain, popping, or a catching feeling in the finger or thumb. When the tendon catches, the pulley also becomes swollen and irritated, creating a vicious cycle. Sometimes the tendon becomes stuck in the pulley and the finger can't be straightened or bent.

Trigger finger or thumb often starts with a sense of discomfort at the base of the digit, which may also thicken slightly. If the finger begins to trigger or lock, you may think the problem is at the middle knuckle of the finger or the top knuckle of the thumb, but it's actually inflammation of the pulley at the base of the affected finger. It's not clear what causes trigger finger, but people who are older than 40 and who have rheumatoid arthritis, gout, or diabetes seem to be more susceptible to the problem.

Wearing a splint, taking anti-inflammatory drugs, and getting a steroid injection in the area around the tendon can all help break the cycle of inflammation and pain. If your symptoms don't improve, surgery is an option. The operation opens the pulley, allowing the tendon to glide through it more easily—a quick procedure that takes only about 10 minutes. Usually, this restores finger movement right away, although some people feel tenderness, swelling, and discomfort for four to six weeks, or possibly longer. A full recovery, meaning your finger feels back to normal, often takes at least three months and can take up to a full year.

> **Symptoms of trigger finger (or thumb)**
> ✔ Pain and sometimes swelling where the finger or thumb joins the palm
> ✔ When you bend or straighten the affected digit, it may catch and then suddenly release

> **Symptoms of tennis elbow**
> ✔ Pain on the outer side of the elbow and down the forearm, usually in your dominant arm
> ✔ Worsening of pain if you straighten your wrist or try to pick up a heavy object

Tennis elbow

Why include tennis elbow in a report on hands? Also known as lateral epicondylitis or lateral elbow tendinopathy, this condition involves degenerative changes of the fibers that attach your forearm muscles to the outside of the elbow. These muscles lift the wrist and hand. So, every time you use your hand, the tendon attached to your elbow hurts. You may feel mild pain in your outer elbow that gradually worsens over weeks and months, becoming a severe, burning pain. Pressing the outside of the elbow or lifting even very light objects, like a book or coffee cup, can hurt.

Although the problem can occur in people of all ages, it's most common between the ages of 30 and 50. Despite the name, most people with tennis elbow don't play tennis or other racquet sports. They may be involved in work or other activities that require them to use their forearm muscles in repetitive, vigorous ways—shoveling snow, for example. But some have no apparent reason for developing symptoms.

Treatment focuses first on easing pain. Reducing activity and putting ice on your elbow can help; so can anti-inflammatory medications. Your doctor or hand therapist may also recommend certain braces or splints that allow your tendons and muscles to rest and heal (see "Splints," page 25). Kinesiotape (see page 26) is an increasingly popular option. Massage and other soft-tissue techniques and pain-free stretching and strengthening exercises may be added to your regimen as your treatment progresses. The exercise program may also include strengthening of your shoulder and core to improve your overall mobility and function.

Your symptoms should improve within six to eight weeks, although complete healing may take as long as 12 to 15 months. A therapist can teach you specific exer-

Continued on page 26

Splints

The basic purpose of a splint is to immobilize an injured or inflamed part of the body, allowing it to heal. Splints can provide pain relief, allow you to function, or realign your joints to a more anatomically correct position. Certified hand therapists are specifically trained to assess your hand and choose or fabricate a splint to meet your needs.

Splints come in a wide range of materials and forms. Prefabricated splints from the drugstore or a medical supply store (such as splints 2 and 3—the MetaGrip and Cool Comfort, respectively) work well to restore function for people with arthritis of the CMC joint of the thumb, provided you choose and adjust the splint correctly. Other conditions require specially fabricated splints, which are usually made of thermoplastic materials and molded to fit around the contours of your hand (splints 1, 4, and 5). Silver ring splints, which look like jewelry, are flexible and strong and can be worn on the fingers during most activities to treat trigger finger and various other problems in thumb and finger joints (splint 6). These splints are ordered after you are measured by a hand therapist. Less expensive finger splints are available in other materials and are fitted and issued to the patient by the hand therapist. For people with rheumatoid arthritis, resting hand splints keep joints in a neutral position to prevent muscle shortening and joint deformity (splint 7).

Static splints (all seven shown here) hold a joint in one position. Dynamic splints (not pictured) do not. Some are designed to help lengthen tightened joint capsules, muscles, and tendons. Others, which feature elastic or spring-loaded parts, provide for missing motion in the hands and wrists caused by muscle weakness or nerve damage.

Of course, a splint only works if you have the right type for your specific problem and if you use it correctly. For example, splints used to treat carpal tunnel syndrome (splint 4) are intended to be worn only when you're sleeping or resting—not when you're using your wrist. Some common complaints about splints are that they don't look good, they immobilize too many joints (which limits your ability to function), or they fit poorly (which can cause pressure and irritate the skin). If you're experiencing any of these problems, consult a therapist for guidance.

A short opponens splint, used when the hand is at rest, immobilizes the thumb only and can help ease osteoarthritis of the thumb.

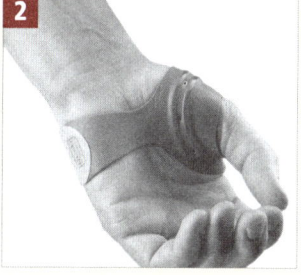

A semi-rigid splint rests the base of the thumb to ease osteoarthritis, but allows for light to moderate function.

A soft functional splint provides gentle support to the thumb and still allows you to use your hand for light activities.

A wrist immobilizer holds the wrist straight, in a neutral position, which helps people with carpal tunnel syndrome. It is used when the hand is at rest. To treat tennis elbow, this type of splint may also be configured with the wrist tilted up to reduce tension on the extensor tendons.

A long opponens splint, often recommended for de Quervain's tenosynovitis, immobilizes both the thumb and wrist. It is used when the hand is at rest.

A silver-ring splint blocks hyperextension of the middle joint of the finger to correct a swan-neck deformity.

A resting hand splint, sometimes recommended for rheumatoid arthritis, aligns the fingers to prevent ulnar deviation.

Continued from page 24

cises to strengthen the affected muscles and tendons, and show you how to modify your activities so your symptoms don't return. Most people are completely cured with these treatments. But one in 10 patients ends up needing surgery to remove damaged tendon tissue and reattach normal tendon tissue to bone.

Golfer's elbow

You can also develop degenerative changes on the inside of your elbow; this is known medically as medial epicondylitis. This condition usually arises from movements that involve turning the arm down and flexing the wrist, such as during a golf swing, which is why it's also known as golfer's elbow. But any activity that requires you to repeatedly bend your wrist or grip, grab, and turn your hand can cause the condition. The symptoms include tenderness and pain in the inner elbow, which worsen if you bend your wrist. The treatments resemble those for tennis elbow, but focus on the inner elbow.

> **Symptoms of golfer's elbow**
> ✔ Pain and tenderness in the inner elbow
> ✔ Worsening of pain if you bend your wrist

Dupuytren's disease

This uncommon hand problem is also known as Dupuytren's contracture because it causes the fingers to slowly contract and curl toward the palm. It results from an abnormal thickening of the fascia—the tissue between the skin and tendons—in the palm. Some people develop a tough cord beneath the skin stretching from the palm to the fingers, which prevents the fingers from fully straightening (see Figure 9, page 27).

Although no one knows exactly what causes Dupuytren's disease, it's almost certainly inherited. Named after the French surgeon who first treated the disease in 1830, Dupuytren's mostly affects people with Northern European heritage and is more common in men than women. Cigarette smoking, epilepsy,

Kinesiotape

You may have noticed athletes sporting colorful tape in various designs on their skin. Kinesiotape is thin, stretchy cotton tape with latex-free adhesive. Your therapist can show you how to use the tape, applied in a specific pattern, as an adjunct to your exercise program and hands-on therapy. It can reduce pain and swelling via stimulation through the skin, decrease spasms by helping muscles to relax, support muscles and joints without reducing your range of motion, lessen pressure on injured areas in between treatments, and help you sense when you are keeping your arms and hands in proper alignment. On the wrist and hands, therapists often use kinesiotape in therapy for such problems as tennis elbow, De Quervain's tendinitis, and finger sprains. A certified hand therapist can assess if kinesiotape would be beneficial to you and teach you how to properly apply it to get the desired benefits.

and diabetes may increase the risk for Dupuytren's.

The condition often begins with a small lump or pit in the palm, usually near the crease of the hand, closest to the base of the ring and little fingers. Dupuytren's disease usually doesn't hurt, but the initial nodules in the palm may be painful. Still, you may not notice the problem until you cannot flatten the palm of your hand on a table or other flat surface, which may not happen for months or even years. In a poem published in *The Journal of the American Medical Association*, a physician affected by the disease described his father's (and his own) experience with the deformity. He was "puzzled by the stinging and the curl of his fingers about a phantom hardball caught barehanded." In severe cases, when the fingers contract into the palm, it's difficult to do everyday activities such as washing your hands, putting on gloves, and stuffing your hands in your pockets. With Dupuytren's, it's impossible to straighten the fingers, unlike a trigger finger, which can be intermittently straightened. Often both hands are affected.

In the past, people with Dupuytren's disease were usually treated with surgery to release their bent fingers. Afterward, patients wore splints to keep their fingers straight, followed by therapy to ease swelling and help them regain finger function. But the thickened fascia and cord characteristic of this disease sometimes returned in the same place or elsewhere in the hand. That's also the case for a less-invasive procedure called needle aponeurotomy or percutaneous fasciotomy, in which the doctor uses a small needle to divide and sever the contracting bands in the palm. The procedure is done under local anesthesia. People usually recover quickly, returning to normal activities within just a few days, without needing bandages or splints. However, despite the initial high success rate, the condition returns in up to 65% of people.

In 2010, the FDA approved a nonsurgical treatment for Dupuytren's disease. Marketed under the name Xiaflex, the drug is made from an enzyme, called collagenase clostridium histolyticum, which breaks down the collagen fibers causing the contracture. A doctor injects the medication directly into the collagen cord in your hand. Several days later, your hand is numbed and manipulated to release the cord (see Figure 10, below). Over the following four to eight weeks, you wear a splint at night that straightens your finger, and you perform exercises several times a day to maintain your finger's range of motion. The most common side effects include swelling, bleeding, and pain in the injected area. In

Figure 9: Anatomy of Dupuytren's contracture

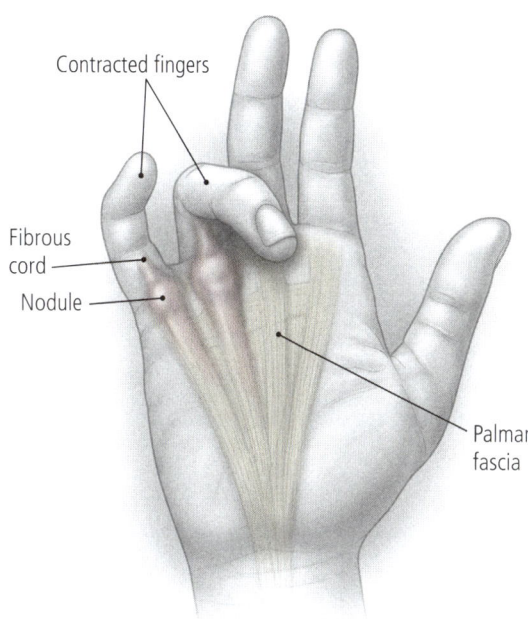

A contracture from Dupuytren's disease develops when the palmar fascia (the tissue overlying the tendons in the palm) shortens and contracts, pulling the fingers inward. The first sign may be a nodule near the crease of the hand below the finger. A fibrous cord may develop that extends from the palm to the finger.

▸ **Symptoms of Dupuytren's disease**
- ✔ Small lump or pit in the palm crease closest to the ring and little fingers
- ✔ Inability to flatten the palm on an even surface
- ✔ Fingers may eventually curl toward the palm

Figure 10: Before and after collagenase treatment of Dupuytren's contracture

At left, severe contractures of the ring and middle fingers in a person with Dupuytren's disease before treatment with injectable collagenase (Xiaflex). At right, the same hand after treatment.

Photos reprinted with permission, Barry P. Simmons, M.D.

rare cases, the collagenase can leak into the tendon, causing it to rupture—a serious complication.

In a study published in *The New England Journal of Medicine*, 308 people with contractures of 20° or more in the MCP or PIP joint of the ring or little finger received injections of either Xiaflex or a placebo. The following day, the investigators manually extended the fingers (as much as the patients could tolerate) to break the cord and release the contracture. Subjects could receive up to three injections (at intervals of about one month). Nearly 85% of joints injected with collagenase showed some improvement, compared with 12% of those receiving placebo injections. On average, Xiaflex improved range of motion by 37°, compared with a 4° improvement in those who got a placebo injection. Other studies show that after two years, recurrence rates were 14% for MCP joints and 23% for PIP joints.

A larger study that included 924 treated joints in nearly 650 people reported a success rate of 67% after three years. Success was defined as close to a full extension of the fingers, or a contracture of 5% or less following treatment. Many other people had less dramatic but still noticeable improvements in their contractures. That's likely why even though just over a third of the procedures were deemed "unsuccessful," only 7% of the participants had a repeat procedure.

Although all the treatments for Dupuytren's contracture are beneficial, none cure the disease. Three years after Xiaflex, recurrence is about 45% at the MCP joint and 65% at the PIP joint. However, repeat injections are possible.

Ganglion cysts

If you notice a small, firm lump on the back of your wrist or hand, don't be alarmed. Chances are it's a ganglion cyst, a common, harmless growth that develops from inside a joint, like a tiny balloon on a stalk (see Figure 11, at right). The balloon may be filled with fluid or a jelly-like substance and can usually be felt underneath the skin. The cyst may be painful and may wax and wane in size, sometimes growing as large as a peach pit. Aside from the back of the hand, ganglion cysts can also form on the underside of the wrist, between the thumb and the pulse point, or at the base of a finger. An old-time treatment for these cysts was to hit them with a heavy book, which is why they're also known as "Bible cysts." Don't try this, however—it's not effective, and you could fracture your wrist!

▶ Symptoms of ganglion cyst
- ✔ Small, firm lump on the hand that is usually painless, ranging in size from a pea to a peach pit
- ✔ Lumps may disappear and reappear

Figure 11: Ganglion cyst

A ganglion cyst on the top side of the wrist.

It's not clear what triggers most ganglion cysts, although it is thought that flaws in the synovial lining of a joint allow the synovial fluid to form a fluid-filled cyst that can change shape. They're more common in women than in men, and gymnasts (who often put a great deal of pressure on their wrists) seem to be especially susceptible to them.

Often, these cysts simply disappear with time. But if the cyst is painful, affects your daily activities, or is unattractive, you may want to consult a doctor. To diagnose the condition, the doctor will probably press on the cyst to check for tenderness or hold a penlight up to the cyst to see if the light shines through.

Because activity can cause the cyst to hurt, you may be advised to wear a wrist splint (see photo, page 31) to relieve symptoms. After any pain or discomfort subsides, wrist-strengthening exercises may help (see "Exercises for the hands," page 43). Your doctor can also aspirate the cyst, which involves numbing the area and puncturing the cyst with a needle to draw out the fluid. But the cysts nearly always recur after aspiration. If the entire cyst is surgically removed, recurrence rate is about 10%. The surgery involves removing part of the affected joint capsule or tendon sheath. Recovery time varies, but you should be able to return to your daily activities within two to six weeks.

Carpal tunnel syndrome and other "pinched" nerves

Three major nerves travel from the spinal cord all the way to the hand: the median, ulnar, and radial nerves. Each is housed within passageways or tunnels, which may become narrowed for a variety of reasons. When that happens, it puts pressure on the nerve, causing symptoms such as weakness, tingling, or numbness in the hand.

The best-known and most common of these trapped or pinched nerve problems is carpal tunnel syndrome, which affects the median nerve as it passes through the wrist to the thumb, index, and middle fingers, and the thumb side of the ring finger (see Figure 12, at right). A similar but far less common problem, known as cubital tunnel syndrome, occurs with compression of the ulnar nerve, which passes through the inner part of the elbow. Other nerves can also become entrapped, but instances of this are very rare.

Carpal tunnel syndrome

The carpal tunnel consists of a U-shaped cluster of eight bones at the base of the palm. A strong ligament, called the transverse carpal ligament, arches across the bones, forming the roof of the tunnel. Within this tunnel lies the median nerve, which controls sensations in the palm side of the thumb, the index and middle fingers, and half of the ring finger. It also transmits the impulses to certain hand muscles that allow the fingers and thumb to move. If the carpal tunnel narrows, the resulting pressure decreases the blood supply to the nerve, causing carpal tunnel syndrome.

The classic symptoms are pain, weakness, and tingling in the thumb and affected fingers. Often, these symptoms occur at night and awaken you from sleep. Sleeping with the wrists flexed—a common habit—can contribute to the nighttime symptoms. After you awaken, you may need to shake your hand to restore normal feeling. Some people say their hands feel swol-

Figure 12: Nerve entrapment in carpal tunnel syndrome

A. Neutral

B. Flexion

C. Extension

A feeling of numbness, tingling, or weakness in the fingers is often the result of nerve entrapment, a narrowing of the passageway or "tunnel" that the nerves must pass through to reach the hand. In this illustration, for example, the median nerve passes freely through the carpal tunnel when the hand is in a neutral position **(A)**. But when the hand is flexed **(B)** or extended **(C)**, the tunnel is narrowed, pressing on the nerve and causing symptoms in people who are susceptible to this condition.

len and useless, even though their hands don't appear swollen. As the condition progresses, you may start to feel tingling during the day, and the pain may radiate up your arm. It may become difficult to make a tight fist, grasp small objects, or do other things with your hands. In severe, chronic cases, persistent numbness may occur, and the muscles at the base of the thumb may weaken. You may even lose the ability to distinguish between hot and cold by touch.

Carpal tunnel syndrome affects about 3% of working adults. Women are three times as likely as men to have carpal tunnel syndrome, and the condition is most common in women ages 50 to 55. It is not clear why some people get carpal tunnel syndrome and others don't. However, the following factors may contribute to the condition:

Heredity. Experts estimate that genes account for about half of cases. That assessment is based in part on studies that show a much higher risk in women who have an identical twin with the disorder compared with those with a fraternal twin. (Identical twins have all of the same genes, while fraternal twins have fewer genes in common.)

Tunnel size. Although the size of your wrist doesn't seem to matter, having a smaller carpal tunnel may make you more prone to the problem. This may help explain why women are more likely than men to develop carpal tunnel syndrome.

Diseases. Metabolic diseases (such as diabetes and thyroid disease) and autoimmune diseases (such as rheumatoid arthritis, lupus, and connective tissue disorders) have been linked to a higher risk of developing carpal tunnel syndrome.

Previous bone dislocation or fracture. These injuries may cause bones to protrude into the carpal tunnel, narrowing it.

Hormone status. Approximately 20% of pregnant women develop carpal tunnel syndrome during their last trimester, most likely because of fluid retention caused by hormones. Symptoms usually disappear gradually after the baby is delivered. Having your ovaries removed (surgical menopause) also appears to increase the risk.

Body weight. Being overweight or obese appears to raise the risk—perhaps as much as twofold.

Wrist position. Keeping your wrists bent while sleeping, reading, or driving may contribute to carpal tunnel syndrome.

Occupation. Multiple excellent studies dispel the notion that carpal tunnel syndrome stems from computer use or repetitive motion. Occupations that have been linked to carpal tunnel syndrome involve the use of power tools, especially in a cold environment. For example, meatpackers who use chain saws in a refrigeration locker are prone to the problem, as are workers in the logging industry. However, these cases are most often seen in younger men. There also appears to be an association in these occupational groups between carpal tunnel syndrome and workplace-related Raynaud's syndrome, which is also linked to the use of vibrating tools.

Diagnosing carpal tunnel syndrome

Your doctor will ask you to describe your symptoms and to recall when, how often, and how severe they are. He or she will examine your hands, arms, shoulders, and neck to determine whether the complaints might be related to daily activities and rule out other conditions that might mimic carpal tunnel syndrome. Routine laboratory tests, including x-rays and blood tests, which can reveal diabetes, arthritis, and fractures, may also be done. The doctor will examine your wrists and hands for signs of tenderness and swelling and test the sensation in each finger. He or she will also assess the muscles at the base of your hand to see if they show signs of weakness.

In addition, doctors use specific tests to try to elicit the symptoms of carpal tunnel syndrome. In the Tinel test, the doctor taps or presses on the median nerve. If that causes tingling in the fingers or a shock-like sensation, the test is positive, meaning you may have carpal tunnel syndrome. The modified Phalen, or

> ### Symptoms of carpal tunnel syndrome
> ✔ Pain, weakness, tingling, and numbness in the thumb, index and middle fingers, and half of the ring finger, especially at night
> ✔ Difficulty making a fist, grasping small objects, or doing other manual tasks

wrist-flexion, test involves holding the elbows straight and flexing the hands and wrists. This test is positive if your fingers tingle or feel numb after one minute.

You may need additional tests to confirm the diagnosis. One is a nerve conduction test (also called a nerve conduction velocity or NCV test), which uses a machine that administers weak electric shocks via small electrodes placed on the hands and wrist. The electrodes measure how quickly the nerves are able to transmit impulses. In another test known as electromyography, the clinician inserts into the muscle a fine needle that measures electrical activity, which reveals the severity of any damage to the median nerve.

More recently, ultrasound has been used to confirm the diagnosis. This is a noninvasive procedure that causes no pain..

To determine how compressed your median nerve may be, and whether it is interfering with sensation in your hand enough to place you at risk for burning or cutting yourself, a clinician may measure your ability to feel the pressure from being poked with a strand of nylon (called the Semmes-Weinstein monofilament exam). In addition, he or she may test the shortest distance you can detect between two points on your hand being touched.

Treating carpal tunnel syndrome

If you have underlying health problems that may be contributing to carpal tunnel syndrome, such as diabetes or arthritis, they should be diagnosed and treated for your overall health.

Self-help. It's important to rest the affected hand for at least two weeks, avoiding any activities that make your symptoms worse. Because bending the wrist down or up can make symptoms worse, it can help to wear a splint that keeps your wrist in a neutral position. Many people find that wearing a splint at night is an effective treatment, especially if they tend to flex their wrists during sleep, as many people do.

Medications. There's no evidence that ordinary NSAIDs such as aspirin, ibuprofen, and naproxen are effective for treating carpal tunnel syndrome. The same goes for the COX-2 inhibitor celecoxib (Celebrex). On rare occasions, some doctors prescribe corticosteroid pills, but these shouldn't be taken for

This is one of many brands of prefabricated wrist splints for carpal tunnel syndrome. It keeps the wrist in a neutral position, while allowing the fingers and thumb to move freely. Consult a hand therapist to help you choose and adjust your splint. Wear it only at night. This splint can also be used for a ganglion cyst.

more than one or two weeks, and people with diabetes should not take them at all.

Hand therapy. Hand therapy for carpal tunnel syndrome focuses on decreasing the pressure on the median nerve in the carpal tunnel and increasing circulation to the area. It is most effective if it takes place before symptoms are severe. The therapist will work with you on ways to treat the problem, such as wearing a splint at night, adapting tools to lessen vibrations, pacing or rotating tasks at work, and learning how to keep the wrist in a neutral position during activities. Gentle hand exercises may or may not be prescribed, depending on your situation. Avoid squeezing a therapy ball or sponge, as it will not help with carpal tunnel syndrome and may only worsen the condition. Specific tendon-gliding exercises may be suggested to relieve pain and tingling by improving the way your tendons move through the carpal tunnel, but these can irritate the nerve and need to be done cautiously and under the guidance of a therapist. If you have constant numbness or atrophy of your thumb muscles, you should be evaluated by a hand surgeon.

Injections. Corticosteroid injections into the carpal tunnel may relieve symptoms, especially in younger people who have had symptoms only for a short time. Studies on the long-term benefits of steroid injections have had mixed results; for most people, pain returns within two to four months.

Surgery. Many people improve with one or more of the above treatments. However, if you have persistent numbness and pain, have trouble gripping or grasping things, or are losing muscle mass in your thumb, surgery may be the right choice for you. Usually, it is recommended only if your symptoms last longer than six months. However, people older than 65 may benefit from earlier treatment, because their symptoms tend to progress more quickly and be more debilitating.

The goal of surgery is to create more space in the tunnel by releasing the transverse carpal ligament, which relieves pressure on the median nerve. Many procedures are done using local anesthesia and don't require an overnight hospital stay. There are two basic approaches to carpal tunnel release—open and endoscopic—plus a variation on the first called small palmar incision surgery, or the "mini-open."

- **The traditional, or open, procedure** consists of making an incision up to two inches long in the hand and wrist to enlarge the carpal tunnel. This technique has the advantage of allowing the surgeon to see the anatomy of your wrist clearly, which lessens the risk for injury to nearby nerves and other vital structures. But with open surgery the scar is more likely to be tender, and the recovery period slightly longer, compared with the endoscopic technique.
- **Endoscopic surgery** involves making one or two smaller (half-inch) incisions in the wrist and palm.

Help for computer-related hand problems

If you work in an office, it's a good idea to have an ergonomic evaluation of your workspace to avoid habits that may put you at risk for a variety of musculoskeletal disorders. If that's not possible, the following tips may help:

- Keep your wrists in a neutral position, not flexed downward or extended upward, when using your computer. To check, place your forearm and hand, palm facing down, on a flat, hard surface with your wrist straight. Put a Band-Aid lengthwise over the top of your wrist, and then move to your keyboard and type. If the Band-Aid stretches or goes slack, your wrists aren't in a neutral position.
- Get up from your desk and stretch at least once every hour. In between, take shorter breaks from continuous typing (every 10 or 20 minutes) to rest your hands, palms up, on your lap or on a wrist rest. You can set a smartphone reminder or install software on your computer that reminds you to take micro-pauses or rest breaks and restricts your daily time on the computer.
- Avoid the use of a laptop computer. A desktop model with a detached keyboard is a better solution, as it puts less strain on the hands and wrists. Also, be skeptical about keyboard configurations (such as split keyboards) or mouse designs claiming to be ergonomic. It will take many years of study to learn whether such changes translate into fewer work-related upper-extremity musculoskeletal disorders.
- Do not use splints or anti-inflammatory medicine that will you allow you to type more, because this may make the problem worse. Instead, use splints at night when you are resting.
- See a hand therapist to learn exercises and stretching techniques to ease discomfort.

Ergonomics specialists who design strategies to improve the fit between workers and their jobs suggest the following arrangement for computer workstations:

- Keep documents, telephone, keyboard, mouse, and supplies within easy horizontal reach—not more than 16 to 18 inches away.
- Place the computer monitor directly in front of you, at arm's length, with the top line of the screen at or slightly below eye level (possibly lower for someone with bifocals or trifocals).
- Set your keyboard on an adjustable tray so that your forearms are parallel to the floor, wrists are straight and in line with your forearms, and elbows are relaxed and bent at a 90° angle at your waist.
- Keep your mouse close to the keyboard at the same height so that your elbow stays by your side.
- Consider using voice-activated computer programs.
- Use an adjustable chair, with a rounded front edge and good lower- and upper-back support, positioned so that your knees are slightly lower than your hips, and your feet rest firmly on the floor (or on a footrest).

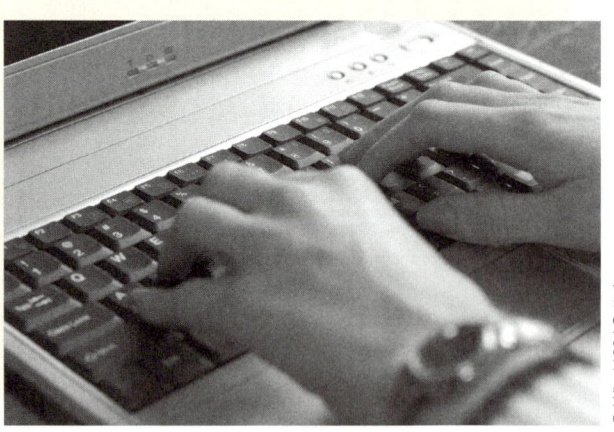

The surgeon inserts a tiny camera attached to a slender tube (endoscope) through one incision, views the tissue on a screen, and uses tiny surgical tools placed through an incision to cut the carpal ligament. Smaller incisions minimize scarring and speed recovery by up to two weeks. However, endoscopic surgery has a higher risk for complications, such as damage to the median or ulnar nerve.

- **Small palmar incision surgery**, a newer technique, involves a one-inch incision in the middle of the palm. The idea is to keep the incision small enough to avoid a long recovery, but large enough that the surgeon can see clearly and avoid injuring any nearby tissues. This procedure is also known as a "mini-open" technique because it does not use an endoscope. Recovery time is similar to that for the endoscopic procedure.

Most surgeons prefer one technique over the others. Many feel that the risks involved with the endoscopic technique—although extremely low—aren't worth the improvement in recovery time, which averages only about a week. However, if a faster recovery is vital to doing your job or other important activity, the endoscopic procedure can be a good choice. It's also worth noting that the "mini-open" technique leaves only a very small scar, hardly bigger than those from the endoscopic technique.

Success rates for these surgeries are high, with 80% to 90% of people reporting relief of daytime and nighttime symptoms after six weeks. But people vary significantly in how quickly they recover. You can expect to resume your strength more gradually, and it may take a year or two before you feel you're back to normal.

Researchers at Harvard's Brigham and Women's Hospital (led by Dr. Barry P. Simmons, the medical editor of this report) conducted a 13-year follow-up of people who received the mini-open surgery. Eighty-eight percent of the 113 people who responded to the survey said they were completely or very satisfied with the results. Asked about their current symptoms, 87% reported good results, and fewer than 2% needed repeat carpal tunnel surgery. In addition, the complication rate in this group was near zero.

Yoga. In one small study, people with carpal tunnel syndrome who took twice-weekly yoga classes for two months had less pain and better grip strength than those who used wrist splints or no treatment.

Hand dystonias: Writer's cramp and musician's cramp

Writer's cramp, a rare condition characterized by an abnormally tight grip on the pen and awkward hand, wrist, and elbow positions, is sometimes mistaken for repetitive strain injury. But it's actually a form of dystonia, a neurological problem that results in sudden, involuntary muscle contractions.

So-called focal dystonias are localized to a particular part of the body and can affect muscles in such places as the neck, eyelids, and vocal cords. They usually occur only in people who assume abnormal positions for long time periods, and only when they perform specific tasks. In adults, focal dystonia of the hand is perhaps the best known, although it accounts for only a tiny fraction of hand conditions. Writer's cramp (also called musician's cramp) is a spasmodic contraction of the muscles of the hand and forearm. The fingers may suddenly freeze up, dramatically affecting the ability to write or play an instrument. Some golfers experience hand dystonias while putting, a phenomenon that's been nicknamed "the yips."

These uncommon afflictions are thought to stem from abnormal functioning of a deep brain structure called the basal ganglia. The basal ganglia initiates and controls the body's movements. Researchers believe that an imbalance of the neurotransmitter dopamine may underlie some forms of dystonia. As with many medical conditions, anxiety and stress—common among professional musicians and athletes during performances—seem to make the problem worse.

Several medications used to treat Parkinson's disease, including trihexyphenidyl (Artane) and benztropine (Cogentin), have been tested for writer's cramp, but the side effects usually aren't worth the small benefit. Another treatment that's gained interest is the injection of botulinum toxin type A (Botox), a substance best known for its cosmetic use to erase wrinkles in the face. A study in the journal *Neurology* found that 69% of musicians with musician's cramp were helped by the injections. A review of studies on the use of botulinum toxin injections to treat writer's cramp found that 50% to 70% of patients were helped. Muscle weakness was a common side effect, both in those who got relief from their cramps and in those who did not.

However, there are no high-quality research trials to confirm this finding, and yoga poses that place the wrist in extreme positions may aggravate the condition, especially if done improperly. If you try this option, find a well-qualified instructor who knows about anatomy and can help you make adjustments to the poses as needed—for example, placing weight on the entire forearm rather than the wrists and hands. You should not have pain, numbness, or tingling while practicing yoga.

Acupuncture. The evidence that acupuncture relieves the symptoms of carpal tunnel syndrome is encouraging but not convincing, according to an analysis of several small research studies. Acupuncture can be costly, as it is not usually covered by medical insurance, but some people prefer to try this option before resorting to surgery.

Vitamin B_6. Some popular books recommend taking 100 to 200 milligrams (mg) of vitamin B_6 daily to alleviate carpal tunnel syndrome. But not only is there no scientific evidence of any benefit to this practice, it may be dangerous. Doctors have reported several cases of nerve damage caused by excessive vitamin B_6 use for carpal tunnel syndrome. The recommended daily intake of this vitamin is only 1.5 mg for women and 1.7 mg for men after age 50, and the Institute of Medicine has deemed the safe upper limit of B_6 to be 100 mg per day.

Repetitive strain injury

Certain work-related medical conditions that affect the body's upper extremities and the neck fall under the broad category of musculoskeletal disorders and are variously known as repetitive strain injury, repetitive stress injury, cumulative trauma disorder, or overuse syndrome. These conditions are more common in manufacturing, food processing, and other industries where workers carry out repetitive motions.

Prolonged computer keyboard use may also put you at risk for repetitive strain injury. Excessive typing and contracting the forearm and wrist muscles for long periods of time can lead to pain, tenderness, and tingling in the arms and fingers, although there is not a clear source of injury to the muscles and joints responsible for the discomfort. Other factors that can contribute to problems include incorrect positioning of the keyboard and computer mouse, use of a laptop rather than a desktop computer, and sustained use of a computer mouse. Carpal tunnel syndrome is sometimes misclassified as a repetitive strain injury. Carpal tunnel syndrome is not caused by repetitive motion.

Treating repetitive strain injury

Treating repetitive strain injury largely involves easing the tension in your hands, wrists, and forearms. For heavy computer users, the first step is creating a workspace that minimizes awkward postures and arm movements (see "Help for computer-related hand problems," page 32). If better positioning and self-care don't help, you may need to see a therapist. Therapy may include ice, heat, ultrasound, massage, or various exercises and stretches for the hand.

Cubital tunnel syndrome

The ulnar nerve connects the spinal cord to the muscles of the forearm and hand, as well as the skin on the small-finger side of the hand. The nerve passes behind your "funny bone," the bump on the inner side of your elbow, or medial epicondyle. Hitting that spot traumatizes the nerve, triggering a short-lived shock and tingling sensation, which can radiate down to the ring and little fingers.

When you bend your elbow more than 90°, it stretches the ulnar nerve, pushing against the bony canal. Tasks that require you to extend and flex your elbow repeatedly can irritate and inflame the nerve. In some people, the nerve shifts and snaps over the funny bone. Leaning or resting on the elbow for long periods (while driving, for instance) can also put pressure on the nerve; so can holding a phone to your ear. The

> ▶ **Symptoms of cubital tunnel syndrome**
> ✔ Numbness, tingling, or pain in the ring and little fingers
> ✔ Weakness or clumsiness of the hand
> ✔ Sharp, sudden pain on the inner elbow when touched

JONATHAN'S STORY: Coping with multiple performance-related injuries

As a professional cellist, Jonathan, then 30 years old, practiced for three to four hours at a stretch and traveled the world for performances, teaching assignments, and auditions. Then, during his third audition in 10 days, his ring finger gave out when he pressed it on a string, and he left the stage fearing that the career he had worked for since age 3 was about to be lost. This is Jonathan's story:

My primary care doctor thought my symptoms sounded like tendinitis, and he referred me to a physical therapist who treated me for compression of the nerves between my collarbone and ribs. But after five months of not playing my instrument and of wearing generic splints I had bought off the Internet, I wasn't any better. That time was wasted because I didn't have the right diagnosis! When I finally saw a neurologist in the Performing Arts Clinical Program at the Brigham and Women's Hospital, I was found to have many problems, but not the one I had been treated for. My ulnar nerves were entrapped in both arms—a problem known medically as cubital tunnel syndrome. This created the weakness in my fourth and fifth fingers (the third and fourth in cello fingering). I also had tendinitis in my forearms, trigger fingers, Raynaud's syndrome, and "zingers" from inflamed nerve endings in my left fingertips.

The physical and occupational therapists used many modes of treatment, including deep tissue massage, stretching, ultrasound, iontophoresis, heat and cold, joint mobilization of my back, kinesiotape on my forearms and upper back, silicone caps to wear over my fingertips to keep from irritating the nerve endings, compression gloves and sleeves, and three splints to sleep in. They gave me exercises for strengthening and stretching and started me on regular aerobic exercise. Every month the neurologist tested the strength in my hands and watched me play for five minutes to see if that provoked the finger weakness from the ulnar neuropathy. There were times when it was really hard to make the five minutes, or even to play at all.

After three months, the neurologist decided I could start practicing in two-minute intervals three times a day. Two months later, I had to play an important concert but needed steroids and anti-inflammatories to make it through, and that set my treatment back a little.

The neurologist and the occupational therapist recommended several changes to the setup of my instrument, including a lighter bow and cello case, a lower bridge so I don't have to press the strings as hard, a longer nut so the half-steps are closer together, putting New-Skin on my fingertips since I don't have thick calluses to protect the nerve endings, and switching to posture pegs—tuning pegs that don't stick out near my ear so I can play with better posture and easier movement. The posture peg change was an immediate slice of heaven.

There were also a million big surprises about things I was doing wrong in everyday life. Now I've learned to sleep without bending my arms, use earbuds to talk on the phone, limit my computer typing time, put on gloves before going outside instead of letting the Raynaud's syndrome kick in, wear compression sleeves daily, and wear a hand splint when carrying grocery bags so they don't dig into my palms.

Fifteen months after I started being treated at the performing arts clinic, I would say I'm symptom-free, but to stay that way I don't practice more than 30 minutes at a stretch, get weekly massages, take Pilates lessons a few times a week to work on symmetry in my body, and use all kinds of tools, such as moist heating pads, to stay healthy.

Looking back, except for being told to play in a "relaxed" way, I never got advice about how to prevent or deal with injuries. We musicians need to be more like dancers and sportspeople in how we train and play and use our bodies.

---

condition is also sometimes seen in professional musicians such as pianists and violinists (see "Jonathan's story," above). As with carpal tunnel syndrome, your sleep position may aggravate the problem. People with cubital tunnel syndrome often sleep with bent elbows, sometimes with their hands above the head. Injuries are another potential cause of damage to this nerve.

Symptoms of cubital tunnel syndrome include numbness or tingling in the ring and little fingers. Your hands may become weak and clumsy, and you may have trouble straightening your fingers. Touching the elbow may cause a sudden, sharp pain.

To diagnose cubital tunnel syndrome, the doctor will examine your hand and elbow and ask about your daily work and habits. You may also undergo an x-ray, an NCV test, ultrasound, or electromyography.

Treating cubital tunnel syndrome

Most treatment for cubital tunnel syndrome centers on changing the actions that may have triggered the problem. For instance, switching to a headset-style phone and removing armrests from your office chair may help. Avoid leaning on your elbow, keeping your elbow flexed more than 90°, and doing repetitive actions that require you to bend and straighten your elbow. If you sleep on your back with your arms bent over your head, try sleeping on your side with a pillow supporting the entire length of the arm. A hand therapist may recommend that you wear a soft splint at night to keep your elbow straight and alleviate pressure on the nerve while you are sleeping. A soft kneepad from a sports store, worn on the inside of the elbow, may also help. Your therapist will be able to make a recommendation or fabricate an effective splint. Also, medications to reduce swelling may help (see Table 2, page 9).

Soft splint for nighttime use

Usually, four out of five people improve with these conservative approaches. If you don't, your doctor may suggest surgery, such as ulnar nerve release.

Traumatic hand and wrist injuries

Considering how often you use your hands, it's no surprise that these vital structures are frequently injured. One-third of all injuries seen in emergency rooms involve the hands and arms.

Falls are one of the most frequent causes of these injuries. Many sports, from baseball to rollerblading, also put the hands in harm's way. In fact, about a quarter of all athletic injuries affect the hands and wrists. People in motor vehicle accidents often sustain hand and wrist injuries. Power tools or equipment—especially lawn mowers and snow blowers—are yet another source of danger to the digits.

Most hand injuries are sprains or fractures, both of which can cause swelling, pain, and stiffness and may limit your hand mobility.

A sprain occurs when you stretch or partially tear a ligament, usually from a fall, a sudden twist, or an impact that jolts a joint out of its normal position. Contrary to popular belief, a sprain can be as debili-

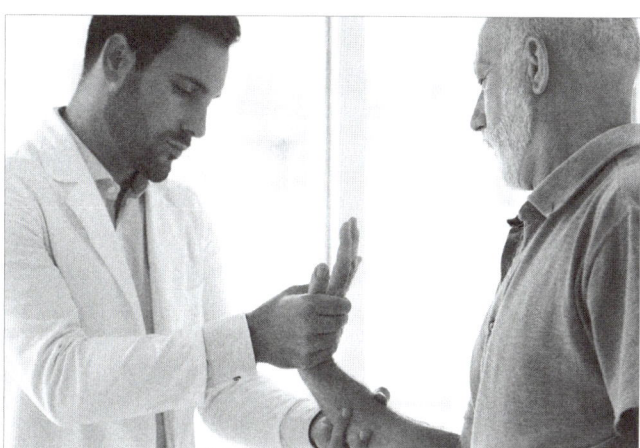

Falls, athletic injuries, and automobile crashes are among the most common causes of sprains, fractures, and dislocations.

tating and painful as a broken bone, or even more so, and it may also take longer to heal. The tendons of the hand are also vulnerable to injury, most often from a cut or a jammed finger, which can tear the tendons away from the bones.

A fracture occurs when a forceful impact breaks the underlying bone. In a simple fracture, the bone pieces remain aligned and stable. In an unstable fracture, the bone is displaced. If the bone shatters, usually from high-energy force, it's known as a comminuted fracture. If a bone fragment has broken through the skin, it is known as an open (compound) fracture. Most bone fractures will heal with time and treatment. However, it may not be possible to save fingers that are severely crushed, mangled, or pierced by a sharp-edged object.

Wrist sprains

Landing on your palm during a fall forces your wrist to bend backward, potentially tearing or stretching the wrist ligaments. In addition to pain and swelling, your wrist may be tender, bruised, or discolored, and you might have felt

Should I see a doctor?

Some sprains are minor and will get better with home treatment that includes RICE (see "First aid: The RICE regimen," page 38), together with pain medications, such as NSAIDs. But other sprains should be evaluated by a health care professional in case you need additional treatment or x-rays to rule out a broken bone. You should consult a clinician if any of the following occurs:

- You have severe pain and cannot put any pressure on the injured joint.
- The injured area looks crooked or has lumps and bumps (other than swelling) that you do not see on the uninjured joint.
- You cannot move the injured joint (note that in some cases you can move the injured area even when a fracture has occurred).
- You have numbness, coolness, or discoloration in any part of the injured area.
- You see redness or red streaks spreading out from the injury.
- You injure an area that has been injured several times before.
- You are in doubt about the seriousness of the injury or how to care for it.

a popping or tearing sensation inside the wrist. The skin may feel warm.

If you have a moderate sprain, you may need to immobilize your wrist with a splint for anywhere from a few days to several weeks, depending on the severity of the injury. A severe sprain can tear the ligament away from the bone, possibly taking a small chip of bone along with it. The resulting injury, known as an avulsion fracture, requires medical care. If you aren't sure about the severity of the injury, see a doctor. Some wrist injuries that feel like sprains may actually be fractures of the scaphoid bone on the thumb side of the wrist (see "Fractures," page 40). Symptoms of a sprained wrist may continue for six to 12 weeks.

Finger sprains, jams, and dislocations

Fingers are susceptible to injury in athletic activities that involve catching a ball, such as basketball, football, baseball, and softball. The treatment depends on the type of injury and whether there has been a dislocation. Typically, the finger is jammed, causing swelling followed by subsequent stiffness of the PIP joint. See your doctor to determine whether there is a dislocation or fracture. If the finger is not dislocated, treatment may involve both ice and taping the finger to the adjoining finger (buddy taping) or splinting. Usually, you can start using the finger within a week or so, but check with your doctor to be sure.

If the finger appears to be deformed, a dislocation likely has occurred. Dislocation requires reduction (putting the bones back in alignment). A dislocation can be so painful that a person will pull on the finger, with a resultant "snap" as the joint goes back in place. In football, a coach may do this to a player, which is why it's called "coach's finger." The person may need an x-ray to check whether the joint is misaligned or fractured. If so, you will need to see a hand surgeon for further treatment, possibly involving surgery. Jammed fingers, with or without dislocation, can be stiff and painful for many months.

If you take a spill on the slopes with your hand strapped to a ski pole, it's easy to sprain your thumb at the MCP joint—a problem known as skier's or ski-pole thumb. The thumb's main ligament stabilizes the MCP joint. If you tear the ligament, you'll lose some or all of your ability to grasp things between your thumb and index finger. You'll also have bruising, tenderness, and weakness.

A partial tear will need to be immobilized in a cast or splint for about four to six weeks. After that, you can start flexion and extension exercises (see "Exercises for the hands," page 43), but continue wearing the splint for protection until the swelling and tenderness go away. If the ligament is completely torn, you may need surgery, after which you'll need to wear a cast for six weeks while it heals.

Tendon injuries

The flexor tendons, which connect the muscles of the wrist and forearm to the fingertips, also control finger movement. Tears or cuts in these tendons make it painful or impossible to bend your fingers.

> ### Symptoms of sprain
> ✔ Pain that develops after an injury, especially if the hand or joint twists or bends at an odd angle
> ✔ Swelling and tenderness of the affected area

First aid: The RICE regimen

If you injure your hand in some way, remember the acronym RICE, which stands for rest, ice, compression, and elevation. These four simple steps will help limit pain and additional damage.

Rest the joint for at least 48 hours.

Ice the injury to minimize swelling, but don't apply the ice directly to your skin. Put cubed or crushed ice in a plastic bag, and then wrap the bag in a towel. You can also use an ice pack, a chemical cold pack, or even a bag of frozen vegetables. Keep the ice on the injured area for no longer than 20 minutes at a time.

Compress the injured area with an elastic compression bandage to provide support and reduce swelling. Wrap it so that it's just slightly snug, taking care not to limit blood circulation.

Elevate your hand above the level of your heart, resting it on a pillow or on the arm of a sofa.

How to prevent falls

1. Make your home environment safer by taking these measures to help fall-proof your house or apartment. (About half of falls happen at home.)
   - Remove things you can trip over (such as papers, books, clothes, and shoes) from stairs and places where you walk.
   - Remove small throw rugs or use nonskid mats or double-sided tape to keep the rugs from slipping.
   - Keep items you use often in cabinets you can reach easily without using a step stool.
   - Install handrails and lights on all staircases.
   - Install grab bars next to your toilet and in the tub or shower.
   - Use nonslip mats in the bathtub and on shower floors.
   - Improve the lighting in your home. As you get older, you need brighter lights to see well. Lamp shades or frosted bulbs can reduce glare.
   - Wear shoes that give good support and have nonslip soles. Avoid slippers or athletic shoes with deep treads.
   - Be especially careful when walking outside in snow and ice. Consider getting special cleats that attach to the soles of your shoes that provide extra traction, such as Yaktrax, and if possible, get someone to support you as you walk.

2. Don't neglect your exercise. Physical activity helps keep your legs strong and improves your balance and coordination, so you can catch yourself if you stumble.

3. Have your health care provider review your medicines, including nonprescription drugs like cold or allergy medications. As you get older, medications may work differently in your body, and certain drugs (and drug combinations) can make you drowsy, potentially leading to a fall.

4. Have your vision checked. If your vision has changed, you may need a new prescription for your glasses. Conditions such as glaucoma or cataracts can also limit vision, increasing your risk for falling.

5. Have your feet checked. Be sure you are wearing footwear that is stable and fits properly, and ask your doctor whether you would benefit from seeing a foot specialist.

▶ **Symptoms of tendon injury**
   ✔ Pain and stiffness following an injury
   ✔ Inability to straighten or bend the affected joint

Figure 13: Mallet finger (baseball finger)

This is a tendon tear caused by a hard blow to the top of the finger. The condition is treated with the use of a splint or small finger cast to immobilize the area for six to eight weeks.

Cuts are the most common cause of these injuries, which can also lead to finger numbness if the nearby nerves are damaged as well. Sports such as football, wrestling, and rugby can also injure these tendons, tearing them from the bone. Since this may happen when one player grabs another player's jersey, catching and pulling a finger, the injury is sometimes known as jersey finger. Repair and rehabilitation of flexor tendons is delicate and precise. The earlier you seek treatment (no more than a week or so after the injury), the greater your chances of a successful repair.

The extensor tendons, which allow you to straighten your fingers and thumb, are just under the skin on the back of your hand and fingers. Because of their location, they can be easily injured, even by a minor cut. If the tip of your finger is hit with enough force that it bends down toward the palm, the tendon can tear. One common cause is a fast-moving baseball, which is why the injury is sometimes called baseball finger (see Figure 13, above). Known medically as mallet finger, this tendon injury can leave the top of your finger near the fingernail red, tender, painful, and slightly swollen. If the tendon is fully detached from the bone, you won't be able to straighten your finger, which will hang down in an abnormal position. Treatment of an extensor tendon tear involves wearing a splint or cast to keep the end joint stable for six to eight weeks.

Cut or torn tendons need to be repaired. You will need to wear a splint for up to two months and see a therapist for advice on special exercises to aid healing and maintain motion.

Fractures

A broken wrist is the most common fracture among people younger than age 65. The popularity of high-velocity sports that require balance, such as snowboarding and rollerblading, has contributed to an increase in hand and wrist fractures. For older folks, accidental falls can break bones in or near the wrist. Each year, about 29% of adults ages 65 and older fall at least once, according to the CDC. (For tips on fall prevention, see "How to prevent falls," page 39.)

When you fall, your natural reaction is to thrust out your hand to keep your body from hitting the ground

Hand transplantation

First successfully performed in 1998 by a team of surgeons in France, hand transplantation involves the transfer of one or both hands from a deceased human donor to a person who has lost a hand or hands from injury, including severe burns. Unlike a heart or kidney transplant, a hand transplant isn't lifesaving. But for people who have lost one or both hands, the procedure is life-renewing, as everyday activities—from using a fork to touching a loved one—become possible again.

The procedure itself is complicated, involving the transfer of skin, muscle, blood vessels, bones, tendons, and nerves. For this reason, hand transplantation surgery can last anywhere from 12 to 16 hours—about twice as long as a heart transplant. All transplant recipients must take drugs that suppress the immune system for the rest of their lives, so their bodies do not reject the transplanted tissue. Improvements in these medications have helped make hand transplants less risky than in the past.

The only mandatory requirements for matching donors with recipients are size and blood type, although gender, race, skin tone, and age are often considered as well.

Worldwide, approximately 29 people had received single hand transplants and 39 double hand transplants by the end of 2017. According to data from the International Registry on Hand and Composite Tissue Transplantation, all of these people gained what's known as protective sensitivity, meaning the ability to discern whether something is hot or sharp, for example. Most recipients also achieved the ability to tell if an object is fuzzy or smooth (discriminative sensation), and most also regained their ability to do most daily activities. Although 88% experienced at least one episode of acute rejection (which can include swelling and bleeding) within the first year, prompt treatment reversed the problem. Other serious side effects included infections, diabetes, and cancer that may result from taking powerful immunosuppressive drugs. Several transplant recipients—including the first one, who received his hand in France in 1998—had to have their new hands removed because of tissue rejection, apparently because they didn't comply with the regimen of antirejection medication. However, improvements in immunosuppressive treatment in recent years have led to greater optimism about the life-enhancing potential of these procedures in carefully selected patients.

To be considered for a hand transplant, you must be between 18 and 60 years old. The time between your hand amputation and the transplant must be more than six months but less than 15 years. You must also undergo extensive tests and evaluations to determine whether you are physically and emotionally equipped for the surgery. After receiving the transplant, you will undergo two years of intensive occupational and physical therapy to help restore near-normal hand function, and of course you will have to take immunosuppressive drugs for the rest of your life.

If you're interested in receiving a hand transplant, you should be aware that hand transplantation is still considered experimental, which means the procedure can only be performed as part of a research study. Currently, 15 centers in the United States have programs, including Johns Hopkins Medical Center, UCLA, the Mayo Clinic, Emory University, the University of Pittsburgh Medical Center, and Harvard-affiliated Brigham and Women's Hospital (BWH). To date the BWH team has done four double hand transplants. The second patient, a 65-year old man who lost both hands (as well as his lower legs) because of a severe bloodstream infection, is now able to do many everyday activities with his newly transplanted hands, including driving a car, swimming, and playing the piano.

too forcefully. On medical charts, doctors refer to the phenomenon with an apt-sounding acronym, FOOSH, which stands for "fall on outstretched hand." What most people refer to as a wrist fracture is actually a fracture of the radius (the main forearm bone) that occurs just above the wrist—a problem known medically as a Colles' fracture. These fractures are common in adults, especially among middle-aged or older women whose bones have been weakened by osteoporosis. If you break your wrist, many doctors recommend screening for osteoporosis, especially if you have other risk factors for the disease, such as being thin and small.

A Colles' fracture causes pain and swelling just above the wrist. A doctor may need to reposition the bone and immobilize the wrist with a splint or cast. Sometimes a fracture cannot be adequately realigned by manipulating the bones into place, and will require surgery. Recovery from treatment for a Colles' fracture may take as long as six to nine months, depending on the severity of the injury. Interestingly, recovery after surgery may be more rapid, sometimes taking as little as three to six months.

If you fall on the back of your hand instead of the palm side, you may have a Smith's fracture, also

▶ Safety tips for using lawn mowers and snow blowers

✔ Read the instruction manual before using.
✔ Never remove safety devices, including shields or switch guards.
✔ Keep the machine in good working order.
✔ Keep children far away from the work area and never allow them to operate these devices.
✔ Keep your hands and feet clear of all moving parts.
✔ Never insert hands or feet to remove debris, grass, or snow from these machines. Use a stick or broom handle to remove obstructions.
✔ Wear protective ear coverings.
✔ After turning off the machine, wait five seconds for the blades to stop moving.
✔ Wear protective boots, goggles, gloves, and long pants when mowing a lawn.
✔ Don't cut wet grass, and be cautious when mowing hills or slopes.
✔ Keep in mind that the rotating blades are spring-loaded and continue to have energy even when stalled. Therefore, when a locking object is removed, the blade will complete its rotation and potentially cause an amputation.

▶ Symptoms of fracture

✔ Pain directly over a bone
✔ Pain, swelling, and deformity that persist even after following the RICE regimen
✔ Inability to move the hand, wrist, or finger

known as a reverse Colles' fracture. This type of fracture displaces the bone toward the inside of the wrist. This uncommon injury often requires surgery to realign the bones.

Another less-common wrist fracture involves the scaphoid bone, also called the navicular bone. One of the eight carpal (wrist) bones that form the carpal tunnel, the scaphoid is a small bone shaped like a cashew on the thumb side of the wrist. Like a Colles' fracture, a scaphoid fracture usually results from a FOOSH. It causes pain and tenderness in the wrist and in the area just below the thumb. Sometimes blood from the fractured bone fills the wrist joint, producing visible swelling.

Although rare, finger fractures also occur during falls or other trauma to the hand. Signs of a broken finger include pain when touching the bone, swelling, and difficulty moving the finger. The finger may be displaced or deformed. Some finger fractures only need to be taped, while others need realignment. More complicated fractures may require surgery, during which the doctor may insert pins and screws to hold the broken fragments in place.

Finger amputations

Most accidental fingertip amputations occur in young children whose fingers are caught in doors and in men in late middle age who are using power tools. As you'd expect, the middle and index fingers are the most vulnerable. Each year, finger amputations from the use of consumer products send an estimated 23,000 people to emergency rooms.

In young children, almost three in four finger amputations result from fingers being jammed or crushed in a door, either in the car or at home. Pinch guards and other safety measures could prevent many of these injuries, experts say. For adults, injuries often occur when a momentary lapse in judgment or failure to follow safety rules, such as wearing proper safety equipment, results in an injury (see "Safety tips for using lawn mowers and snow blowers," page 41).

If you cut your finger, do the following:
- Elevate the injury and apply ice to reduce bleeding and swelling.
- Cover the finger wound with a dry, sterile dressing.
- Immobilize the affected hand and wrist with a short splint, using any stiff material and tape.

If a finger is completely cut off, take these steps:
- Place the severed finger inside a dry, watertight bag and place the bag on ice.
- Bring the finger to the emergency room. Depending on the nature and extent of the injury, a surgeon may be able to reattach the finger.

Exercises for the hands

Therapists recommend specific exercises to treat specific conditions. Some exercises help increase a joint's range of motion or lengthen the muscle and its associated tendons (called a muscle-tendon unit) via stretching; these are helpful for osteoarthritis as well as tennis elbow and golfer's elbow—but not when the joints are inflamed or painful. Other exercises strengthen muscles around a joint to generate more power or to give that specific body part greater endurance. These are helpful for resolving tendinitis and nonpainful arthritis conditions.

The following examples describe some commonly recommended exercises for people with hand and wrist problems. But if you have a painful or debilitating hand, wrist, or arm condition, it's best to get specific exercise recommendations from a therapist, rather than exercising on your own. All exercises should be done slowly and deliberately, to avoid pain and injury. If you feel numbness or pain during or after exercising, stop and consult a therapist.

Range-of-motion exercises

Your muscles and tendons move the joints through arcs of motion, as when you bend and straighten your fingers. If your normal range of motion is impaired—if you can't bend your thumb without pain, for example—you may have trouble doing ordinary things like opening a jar. These exercises move your wrist and fingers through their normal ranges of motion and help to lubricate all the hand's tendons by making them glide through their sheaths. Hold each position for five to 10 seconds. Do one set of 10 repetitions, three times a day.

Wrist extension and flexion
- Place your forearm on a table with your hand off the edge of the table, palm down. You can use a rolled-up towel for padding, if you like.
- Move the hand upward until you feel a gentle stretch.
- Return to the starting position.
- Repeat the same motions with the elbow bent at your side, palm facing up.

Wrist supination/pronation
- Stand or sit with your arm tucked close to your side with the elbow bent to 90°, palm facing down.
- Rotate your forearm, so that your palm faces up and then down.

Wrist ulnar/radial deviation
- Support your forearm on a table on a rolled-up towel for padding or on your knee, thumb upward.
- Move the hand straight up and down.

Thumb flexion/extension
- Begin with your thumb positioned straight out to the side.
- Move the thumb across the palm and then back out to the starting position.

Hand/finger tendon glide
- Start with the fingers extended straight out.
- Make a hook fist; return to a straight hand.
- Make a full fist; return to a straight hand.
- Make a straight fist; return to a straight hand.

Straight hand   Hook fist   Full fist   Straight fist

Strengthening exercises

By holding light weights (1 to 3 pounds) during the first three range-of-motion exercises above, you can begin a gentle strengthening program. Increase the weight gradually over time, making sure you can control the motion while holding the weight within a normal (or recommended) range of motion. Begin with one set of 10. If you don't experience any pain over the following 24 hours, gradually build up to doing two to three sets of 10, as tolerated, exercising every other day. Make sure the exercise is not painful or causing any numbness. Do the exercises slowly and deliberately, holding the positions for a count of 10. Be sure to do these only every other day, because your muscles need to rest for 24 to 48 hours.

Another set of strengthening exercises for healthy hands involves squeezing a cylinder or ball of putty. Therapy putty, available at medical supply stores and other outlets, is a malleable plastic material used to provide different degrees of resistance for hand exercises to improve grip and pinch strength. Start with the softest putty first and advance only if you can do the exercises without symptoms. You should not feel any pain, numbness, or tingling. You may feel some muscle discomfort after exercise, but it should resolve within 24 hours.

If you have any of the hand conditions described in this report, such as trigger finger, carpal tunnel syndrome, arthritis, or de Quervain's tendinitis, consult a hand therapist for an appropriate exercise prescription.

Putty grip
- Roll the putty into a ball.
- Place the putty in your palm.
- Gently squeeze the putty.
- Repeat the sequence 10 times every other day.

Putty key pinch
- Roll the putty into a short, fat cylinder.
- Place the putty between your index finger and thumb.
- Gently squeeze the putty.
- Repeat the sequence 10 times every other day.

Putty three-point pinch

- Roll the putty into a short, fat cylinder.
- Place the putty between the pads of your thumb and your index and middle fingers.
- Gently squeeze the putty between your fingers and thumb.
- Repeat the sequence 10 times every other day.

Stretching exercises

Stretching helps relax stiff, tight muscles and tendons, maximizing the length of the muscle-tendon units in your hands, wrists, and forearms. If you do repetitive tasks, such as typing or gripping gardening tools, you are at particular risk of muscles shortening and becoming tight and painful. Stretching can help counter that problem. These stretches are especially useful for relieving tendinitis and tight forearm muscles, which are common in people who work at computers for long periods of time.

Do these stretches gently, to the point where you feel the stretch but it is not painful. To get the most benefit, do four repetitions of each stretch twice a day, holding the stretch for 15 to 30 seconds each time. Rest for 30 seconds between repetitions.

Wrist extensor stretches

- Begin with a bent elbow.
- With the other hand, grasp the thumb side of the hand and bend your wrist downward.
- To increase the stretch, bend your wrist toward your little finger.
- Repeat the same exercise with a straight arm.

Wrist flexor stretches

- Begin with a bent elbow.
- Grasp the fingers of that hand with the other.
- Pull the hand back gently.
- Repeat the same exercise with a straight arm.

Resisted isometrics

These exercises keep the joint angle and muscle in the same position as they work against an external force, which provides resistance. Hold the position for 10 seconds, and do one set of 10 repetitions once or twice a day.

Isometric wrist extension

- Hold the affected hand palm down, with the opposite hand on top.
- Try to raise the affected hand, but don't allow it to move.

Isometric wrist flexion

- Same as above, but with the palm facing up.

Dynamic isometrics

These exercises—developed by occupational therapist Lori DeMott of Orthopedic One in Columbus, Ohio—help stabilize the CMC joint in the thumb for people with thumb osteoarthritis and also improve pinch strength. Both the thumb and the index finger work together to create pinches, so both need to be strengthened. These exercises require movement, while keeping the CMC joint of the thumb in one position. Do these with your hand resting on a table.

Squeeze the tennis ball as shown in each illustration, not squeezing hard enough to cause pain and using about 40% of your maximum effort. Hold each position for five seconds. Begin with five repetitions in each position and progress to 10 repetitions, every other day, as long as it doesn't hurt. If you also have carpal tunnel syndrome, do not do these exercises unless advised by your hand therapist because it may worsen the condition.

- Gently squeeze and hold the tennis ball. Because this exercise is primarily for thumb instability, make sure the thumb is also pressing into the tennis ball.

- While gently squeezing the ball, lift your index and middle fingers off the ball in a bunny-ears position. The thumb slightly rotates on the ball, reaching toward the little finger.

- Place a rubber band around the tennis ball. Place your index and middle fingers underneath the band as shown. While gently squeezing the ball, lift the index finger up and outward (toward the thumb side).

Dexterity activities

Practicing activities that require quick fine-motor movements of the hands can help counter the loss of dexterity that often occurs with age and in people with nerve compression or osteoarthritis of the hands.

The following provide some good ways to challenge and improve your dexterity:

- Thread buttons or beads onto a thread or ribbon.
- Sort a variety of small objects, such as coins, buttons, or nuts and bolts.
- Shuffle and deal cards.
- Quickly do and undo buttons, snaps, and zippers.
- Work a jigsaw puzzle.
- Rapidly remove and replace small caps and lids from tubes and jars.
- Pick up small objects with your thumb and index finger, then with your thumb and middle finger, thumb and ring finger, and finally the thumb and little finger.

Sensory re-education activities

After surgery involving a nerve, such as surgery to release compression in carpal tunnel syndrome or repair a cut, your doctor may recommend sensory re-education to help you regain the ability to distinguish types and locations of touch on the hands and fingers. In addition to exercises done with a hand therapist, you can work on improving your sensory abilities with these activities:

- Place various coins in your pocket and try to figure out by feel whether you're touching a penny, nickel, dime, or quarter.
- Hide small objects in a bowl filled with rice or dried beans. Reach in and try to identify the objects without using your eyes.
- Attempt to stack objects (such as checkers, coins, or dominoes) with your eyes open, then closed.
- Sort objects (buttons, coins, nuts, and bolts) with your eyes open, then closed.

Getting a grip: Handy gadgets and advice

When your hands hurt, everyday tasks like opening a jar or chopping vegetables can be a stressful ordeal. A combination of lifestyle changes and ergonomic tools can help you cope. When you use utensils and tools with enlarged or extended handles, your joints don't have to work as hard and are protected from excessive pressure and strain. Here are some tools and tips that can make your day a little easier; see "Resources," page 50, for suppliers of some of these assistive devices.

In the kitchen
Gadgets:
- mini chopper
- electric can opener
- jar key opener to release vacuum pressure before trying to unscrew lid
- easy-grip five-in-one opener for cans, bottles, and jars
- small, nonskid gripper mats to increase traction when opening jars and to place under bowls and other items to prevent slippage
- utensils with built-up, padded handles

Vegetable chopper

  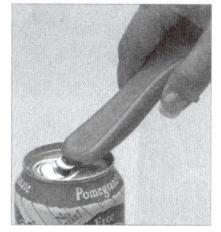

Using the five-in-one device to open a jar, can, or pop-top.

- loop or spring-loaded scissors (for opening packed foods and cutting up foods)
- cheese slicer
- bottle brush for washing cups and glasses
- cookbook stand.

If your hands are severely disabled (for example, from rheumatoid arthritis), you may also want to use these:
- lightweight utensils, pots, and pans
- a rocker knife, which has a curved blade that enables you to cut food on your plate with one hand
- a strap on the refrigerator door (use your arm instead of your hand to pull it open)
- faucet turners at the sink.

General advice:
- Store frequently used items between shoulder and waist level (for example, in utensil holders on the counter).
- Use a steady foot stool to reach higher items.
- Use a rolling cart to move items around the kitchen, and a lazy Susan to improve access to items in cupboards.
- When cooking, avoid a tight grip on utensils.
- Make larger batches of food and freeze extra portions.
- Cook one-pot meals to reduce strain on hands.

Cookbook stand

Rocker knife

Grab bar

In the bathroom
Gadgets:
- electric toothbrush
- pump style toothpaste and soap dispensers
- dental floss holder
- electric razor
- soap-on-a-rope or mitts to hold soap in the shower

- brushes or combs with long handles
- grab bars in the bathtub or shower.

General advice:
- Place your most-used items within easy reach.

In the bedroom
General advice:
- Choose slip-on shoes and loose-fitting garments for easy dressing and undressing.
- Look for clothing with elastic waistbands, large buttons, Velcro fastenings, and zipper pulls.
- Lay your clothes out the night before if you suffer from morning stiffness.
- Fasten your bra in front and turn it around, or choose a front-fastening or pullover style.
- Use a long-handled shoehorn.
- Carry a lightweight purse or briefcase on a strap across your chest or over your shoulder or arm, or consider using a backpack with wide straps or a bag on rolling wheels.
- If you wear jewelry, replace regular clasps with magnetic clasps to make items easier to take on and off.

Velcro fastenings

Button hook

Throughout your home and car
Gadgets:
- key turners
- doorknob turners
- lamp switch adapters
- lightweight vacuum cleaner
- scissors with padded handles or swivel blades (loop or spring-loaded)
- brooms and mops

Key turner

Doorknob extender

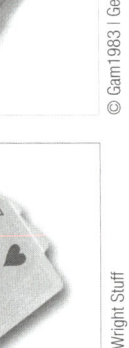
Lamp switch adapter

- with built-up, padded handles
- angled shovels
- phone with automatic dialing
- roller-ball or gel pens and pencils with padded grips
- card holders for playing cards
- car door openers
- padding that provides resistance on the steering wheel
- extended-handle snow removal brush.

General advice:
- When pushing down to stand from a seated position, press with open palms (unless you have wrist problems).
- Strive for good posture; keep your joints in neutral positions.
- If there are no safety concerns, ask your pharmacist to replace childproof caps on your medications.
- Use the eraser end of a pencil to press the keys on your landline phone.
- Don't hold objects (such as a phone) for too long; consider a phone headset.
- Make sure your desk and chair are the correct height for your keyboard.
- When moving heavy items, push rather than pull, and slide rather than lift.
- Spread heavy and light chores throughout the week. Take time to rest!

Padded grips

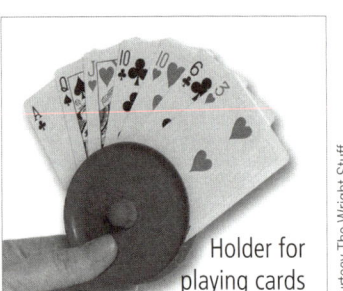
Holder for playing cards

At the grocery store
General advice:
- Buy precut, packaged vegetables and fruits.
- Request paper bags or use recyclable cloth bags, filled with only a few items per bag, and hold them with your forearms facing up, close to your chest.

In the yard and garden

Tool tips:

- Choose lightweight gardening tools that have contoured handles to fit your palm. Pick the right tool for the right job, and keep your tools sharp so they'll work more efficiently.
- Tools with built-up, padded handles can lessen joint strain. Tools with short handles give better control, while those with longer handles offer better leverage.
- Wear gloves to protect your hands from chemicals, sharp items, bug bites, and thorns. Gloves also prevent blisters and can decrease potentially nerve-damaging vibrations from power tools. Lightweight cotton or canvas gloves are best for tasks that don't require protection from mud or moisture. Long, rubber, nonslip-grip gloves both protect and add resistance to the hands, but they make fine-motor tasks more difficult. Gloves with special padding and slight compression designed for people with arthritis (such as Womanswork and Manswork) may be more comfortable and improve your grip.
- Ratcheted tools, like a ratcheting pruner, require less effort to use.
- Look for ergonomically designed tools that allow you to garden while standing up.
- Use carts and tool organizers to keep items within easy reach.
- Use a wheelbarrow for heavy loads.
- Use a coiled hose, which is easier to store.

General advice:

- Maintain good posture. Avoid stooping, and try to maintain the normal curve of your back. Keep your neck straight, your elbows slightly bent, and your wrists in a neutral position (not angled up or down, or deviated to one side).
- Lift with knees bent, back straight, and palms up.
- Keep your loads light.
- Keep objects close to your body, allowing the larger joints to carry more of the load.
- Work below shoulder level and use both of your arms or hands whenever possible.
- Hold objects with a light grasp.
- Take frequent breaks, and rotate tasks. Don't do any single activity for an hour without a break.
- Limit overhead activities to 30 minutes, and stop if you notice any numbness. (Numb fingers are not normal and may be a sign of a compressed nerve, possibly in the upper spine or arm. Consult your doctor to find the cause and pinpoint possible solutions.)
- Don't try to do too much in one day; you'll risk pain and disappointment the following days.

Easy-grip, long-reach fork and cuff

Easy-grip garden tools

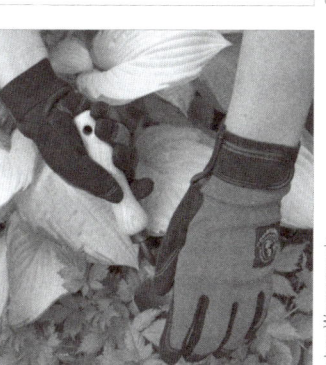
Womanswork digger glove

Resources

Organizations

American Academy of Orthopaedic Surgeons
9400 W. Higgins Road
Rosemont, IL 60018
847-823-7186
www.aaos.org

This nonprofit organization provides education and services for orthopedic surgeons and other health professionals. The website includes patient information and a doctor referral service.

American College of Rheumatology
2200 Lake Blvd. NE
Atlanta, GA 30319
404-633-3777
www.rheumatology.org

This professional organization of physicians, health professionals, and scientists engages in education, research, and advocacy to improve the care of people with arthritis and other rheumatic and musculoskeletal diseases. The website includes patient fact sheets.

American Occupational Therapy Association
4720 Montgomery Lane, Suite 200
Bethesda, MD 20814
301-652-6611
www.aota.org

This professional organization's website offers information for patients, including free 15-minute podcasts about how occupational therapy can help treat a variety of health conditions.

American Physical Therapy Association
1111 N. Fairfax St.
Alexandria, VA 22314
800-999-2782 (toll-free) or 703-684-2782
www.apta.org

This professional organization's website provides a range of information for consumers, including details about therapy for a variety of conditions, an "Ask a PT" feature, and a searchable directory of physical therapists.

American Society for Surgery of the Hand
822 W. Washington Blvd.
Chicago, IL 60607
312-880-1900
www.handcare.org

This professional society provides information for the general public about hand conditions. The website offers a "Find a Surgeon" link.

American Society of Hand Therapists
1120 Route 73, Suite 200
Mount Laurel, NJ 08054
856-380-6856
www.asht.org

This professional organization provides consumer information about common hand conditions and an online searchable index of certified hand therapists.

Arthritis Foundation
1355 Peachtree St. NE, Suite 600
Atlanta, GA 30309
404-872-7100
800-283-7800 (product information; toll-free)
www.arthritis.org

This nonprofit foundation sponsors public education programs and continuing education for professionals, raises money for research, and publishes patient information materials. Local chapters can advise about doctors and sponsor activities such as swimming and self-help classes.

Association for Applied Psychophysiology and Biofeedback
10200 W. 44th Ave., Suite 304
Wheat Ridge, CO 80033
800-477-8892 (toll-free) or 303-422-8436
www.aapb.org

This international society aims to promote understanding and awareness of biofeedback. The website provides information about finding a qualified biofeedback provider (look under the "Consumers" tab).

Hand Therapy Certification Commission
180 Promenade Circle, Suite 300, #41
Sacramento, CA 95834
800-860-7097 (toll-free) or 916-566-1140
www.htcc.org

This professional organization's website includes a link (under "CHT Directory") that allows you to search for a certified hand therapist in your area.

Performing Arts Medicine Association
P.O. Box 117
Englewood, CO 80151
303-808-5643
www.artsmed.org

This professional organization's website includes a link (under "Referrals") that allows you to search for physicians and other health professionals with a special interest in treating musicians.

Products

BraceLab
2615 London Drive
Raleigh, NC 27608
888-235-8221
www.bracelab.com

Braces for the thumb, wrist, and elbow, including the MetaGrip. Have them fitted by a therapist.

Fiskars Brands, Inc.
7800 Discovery Drive
Middleton, WI 53562
866-348-5661 (toll-free)
www.fiskars.com

Hand tools for a variety of uses (crafting, gardening, and doing

Resources *continued*

office work). In any "Products" category, look for the "Easy Action" products, recommended by the Arthritis Foundation.

North Coast Medical, Inc.
8100 Camino Arroyo
Gilroy, CA 95020
800-821-9319 (toll-free) or 408-766-5000
www.ncmedical.com

Occupational and hand therapy products, rehabilitation products for physical therapy, and ergonomic products for the workplace. Products include dressing aids, household helpers, adaptive eating utensils, exercise equipment, transfer devices, and more.

OXO
1331 S. 7th St., 2nd Floor
Chambersburg, PA 17201
800-545-4411 (toll-free)
www.oxo.com

Consumer products designed to make everyday living easier, including the OXO Good Grips line of tools and housewares.

Performance Health
28100 Torch Parkway, Suite 700
Warrenville, IL 60555
800-323-5547
www.performancehealth.com

Rehabilitation equipment and supplies for the professional and the home.

Silver Ring Splints
1140 E. Market St.
Charlottesville, VA 22902
800-311-7028
http://silverringsplint.com

Splints for a variety of conditions, including boutonniere deformity, trigger finger, and swan-neck deformity.

Harvard Special Health Reports

The following reports from Harvard Medical School offer further detail on topics mentioned in this report. They can be ordered by calling 877-648-9457 (toll-free) or by going to www.health.harvard.edu.

Living Well with Osteoarthritis: A guide to keeping your joints healthy
Robert H. Shmerling, M.D., Medical Editor
(Harvard Medical School, 2016)

Rheumatoid Arthritis: How to protect your joints, reduce pain, and improve mobility
Robert H. Shmerling, M.D., Medical Editor
(Harvard Medical School, 2018)

Books

The Hand Owner's Manual: A Hand Surgeon's Thirty-Year Collection of Important Information and Fascinating Facts
Roy Meals
(Virtualbookworm.com Publishing, 2008)

Practical advice for preventing and treating common hand problems such as pinched nerves, broken bones, and arthritic joints, along with tips for keeping your hands healthy.

One-Handed in a Two-Handed World
Tommye-Karen Mayer
(Prince-Gallison Press, 2013)

A step-by-step guidebook for managing just about everything with the use of one hand, whether your one-handedness is temporary, long-term, or permanent.

Glossary

arthritis: Inflammation of a joint, often with destruction of cartilage.

arthrodesis: Fusion of two bones to reduce pain and provide stability to a damaged, arthritic, or painful joint.

arthroplasty: Joint replacement surgery.

autoimmune disorder: A condition stemming from an abnormal immune response generated by the body against its own tissues, cells, or molecules.

Bouchard's nodes: Bony nodules that may form in the middle joints of one or more fingers in people with osteoarthritis.

carpal tunnel syndrome: A condition in which the median nerve is compressed as it passes through a narrow space within the wrist, called the carpal tunnel. It is not caused by repetitive motion, though it may be linked to the use of vibrating tools, such as power tools and chain saws.

carpometacarpal (CMC) joint: Joint where a metacarpal bone of the hand and carpal bone of the wrist come together.

cartilage: A type of connective tissue that protects and cushions the ends of bones.

Colles' fracture: A fracture across the end of the main bone of the forearm, the radius; the most common type of wrist fracture.

crepitus: Grinding sensation or sound when a joint moves.

cubital tunnel syndrome: A condition in which the ulnar nerve is compressed at the elbow.

de Quervain's tendinitis: Inflammation of tendons at the wrist that move the thumb.

distal interphalangeal (DIP) joint: The last joint before the nail on each finger except the thumb; the most common site for osteoarthritis of the hands.

Dupuytren's disease: A condition that causes abnormal thickening in tissues of the hand that forces one or more fingers to curl toward the palm.

dystonia: Abnormal muscle tone or tension in one or more muscles.

epicondylitis: Degeneration of tendons in the elbow, often the result of overuse.

ergonomics: The science of designing and arranging things people use to enable the safest, most efficient interaction between people and things.

ganglion cyst: A benign, fluid-filled cyst commonly found on the back of the wrist or elsewhere on the hand.

gout: Arthritis caused by uric acid crystals.

Heberden's nodes: Bony and fibrous nodules that may form in the end joints of one or more fingers in people with osteoarthritis.

inflammation: A response to injury or foreign invasion designed to protect the body; the symptoms are heat, redness, swelling, and pain.

ligament: A band of fibrous tissue that connects bones and stabilizes joints.

metacarpophalangeal (MCP) joint: The knuckle joint that connects the metacarpal bone in the hand to the finger bone.

mucous cysts: Small cysts that form between the nail bed and the top joint of the finger, most commonly in people with osteoarthritis.

osteoarthritis: A joint disease common with aging, characterized by progressive deterioration of the cartilage that lines the joints; also called degenerative joint disease.

osteophyte: A bony growth on the edge of a joint, usually caused by osteoarthritis; commonly called a bone spur.

phalanges: The finger bones.

proximal interphalangeal (PIP) joint: The middle joint of the finger.

pseudogout: Arthritis caused by crystals of calcium pyrophosphate dihydrate (CPPD) in the joints; also known as calcium pyrophosphate deposition disease, or CPDD.

psoriasis: A skin disease characterized by thickened patches of inflamed, red skin.

pulleys: Rings of connective tissue that form a tunnel for tendons in the fingers, holding a given tendon to the bone.

radial tunnel syndrome: A condition in which the radial nerve is compressed at the elbow.

Raynaud's syndrome: A condition in which the blood vessels in the fingers and other extremities narrow in response to cold or stress, causing them to turn white or blue.

repetitive strain injury: A type of overuse injury caused by repetitive motions, common in manufacturing, food processing, and excessive typing.

rheumatoid arthritis: A chronic autoimmune disorder that causes joints to become painful, inflamed, and sometimes deformed.

scleroderma: A disease of the body's connective tissue that causes the skin to thicken and harden.

sprain: A stretch or incomplete tear in a ligament.

synovectomy: Surgical removal of the synovium.

synovial fluid: A thick fluid that lubricates the joints and tendons.

synovium: A thin membrane that lines joint capsules and produces synovial fluid.

tendon: A tough, fibrous tissue that connects muscle to bone.

tenosynovitis: Swelling and inflammation of the tendon sheath, which decreases the sheath's production of synovial fluid.